Nobody Loves A Farting Princess

Jeni Birr

DEDICATION

This book is dedicated to the best friend I ever had:
my rock, my hero,
my dad.

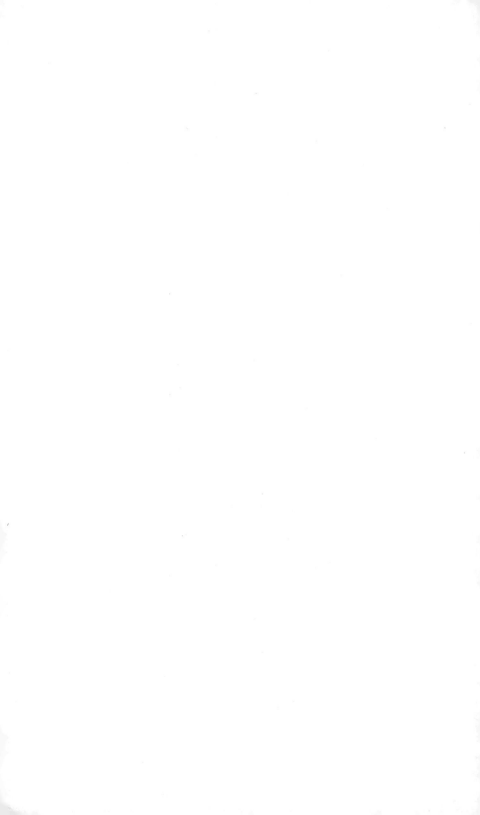

TABLE OF CONTENTS

ACKNOWLEDGMENTS

There are so many people I'd like to thank for turning me into the woman I am today. If we've had any sort of interaction, positive or otherwise, you've impacted me. I like who I am, so I thank each and every one of you for the part you played in my development.

First and foremost: to my parents for bringing me into this world, loving me, supporting me most of the time, and teaching me that I am smarter, prettier, and stronger than I believe. To my brother, Tom, for always providing the comic relief. You may be misunderstood, but I love you. A huge thank you to my grandparents for always being such a tremendous support system on so many levels. To my Uncle Pat, especially for everything you did for my dad a few years back. To my Aunt Jan, you're the coolest aunt a girl could have and your boys are lucky to have you as a mom. To Norm and Karen for being a pretty sweet set of in-laws, and helping us through our tough times. And to the Milton's, for being there for me every step of the way, no matter what I asked.

To my friends growing up: I won't name all of you because that would take some time, but the extra special few are Rob F., Aaron S., Elena L., Nikki D., Sally L., Leah D., Kristen B. and Donnie M. To my educators: particularly Mrs. Klier, Mr. Guilmet, Mr. Inloes, Mr. MacDougall, Mr. Moll, Mr. Williams, Mrs. LaBatt, Mr. Rutherford and especially Mr. "T" Thomas.

To my camp friends: I love you and I miss you. Dave L., Steve "Doc" G., Tom and Andy E., Willie L. and especially you, Lauren R. And to the counselors I probably freaked out: Dan, Dustin, Superman and especially Sandi. I'm truly sorry.

To my Cosi people, my Quiznos people, and my Panera people; for making *almost* every day enjoyable. An extra special thank you to Kristin K. and Lisa L. for throwing us such a wonderful and helpful silent auction. And especially to Steve L. and Chris P. for being so understanding.

To my "Florida" friends: Bob and Kathy T., Rachel E., Nicky L., Carissa B., Michelle W., Jamie H., and Julie S., there is so much I have no idea how I would have made it through without you guys.

To my singer/song-writer/spoken-word/artist people: thank you, each and every one of you for teaching me just how much I love art and music and just how little I know about it. For giving me the inspiration to even pick up a guitar, to start writing songs, to record an EP, and even play a few shows.

To Jeff and Aimee D., Kim S., Corrie L., Brad and Julie E., Ross S. and the rest of my friends I'm drawing a blank on but will certainly kick myself for leaving out, thank you all so much for being such awesome people and such supportive friends.

To Andrea: for being such an amazing friend to me since the day I met you. Thank you for your love, support, hospitality and unwavering friendship. Have a warm coke and a smile, wench.

And lastly, most importantly, to my husband, Eric. We had a very rocky journey to marriage, but it was definitely the best thing either one of us ever did. We are so good for each other. You're an amazing man, a wonderful husband, and I'm pretty sure you saved my life at least a couple times. I love you and thank you, a million times over.

INTRODUCTION

Hello there, lovelies! Let me first take this opportunity to thank you for even beginning this little autobiographical novella. This is the story of my life to date, in all of its grit and minimal glory. It may not be fully accurate, but it is exactly the way I remember it. I have not elaborated, exaggerated or sugar-coated anything. I am well aware that everyone perceives things differently; but this is *my* book, so it's the way I remember it. Is every factoid of my life included? Of course not! But most of what I deem to be relevant is in here, and I'm sure once this is published, I will remember quite a bit that probably should have been in here, but well, what can you do?

Something I believe in pretty fervently, which I try my damndest to uphold, is not speaking poorly of anyone because I don't know their story, what they've been through, or why they're being a royal D.B. (if I feel they're being a royal D.B.); so if I've had beef with anyone, it will not be in here. Several of you just sighed. I heard it. The other thing you should know is that I have a bit of a foul mouth, but I've tried as much as possible to keep the language clean. There are a few (very few,) sections however, where there is need. I apologize in advance.

You will also notice snippets of poems and songs I've written throughout the story. I've been a writer all my life. I wrote my first poem when I was very young and never stopped. Around the age of thirteen, I started writing songs. I'm not saying I'm Maya Angelou or Bob Dylan or anything, but just a heads up if you come across one of these lyrical pearls.

As you've probably already figured out, my style of prose writing is exactly the way I speak, as if I was telling my story to anyone I had known for years, or more likely, someone I had just met that had some time to kill. If this is not your preference, well, then, this is where the S.T.B.Y. rule applies, as one of my favorite mentors used to say: Sucks To Be You.

Please make sure your seat is in its upright position, your tray tables are locked, seatbelt fastened, luggage securely stored below the seat in front of you and all electronic devices are turned off at this time (unless of course you're reading this on an E-reader, those are just fine).

Please enjoy the ride.

CHAPTER 1

I was born 6 weeks early and weighed 5 pounds 5 ounces, at 6:55pm. I'm sure that means something spiritual and sacred, but I'll be damned if I know what it is. I heard my mother tell the story hundreds of times about how she was supposed to be on stage at 7:00, but she didn't make it! And then she would laugh with that cackle of hers that used to embarrass my dad something awful.

I don't really remember much of my childhood. My earliest memory is of kindergarten; getting a gold star for giving Courtney the last piece of pink paper when she started to cry over it, so I went with yellow instead. It just seemed like a nice thing to do. I didn't need pink, yellow was just fine for whatever project we were about to work on, and frankly, I was surprised when I was praised for what I'd done. I've always believed in being kind and not sweating the small stuff. And pretty much all of it, is just that, small stuff.

I do remember having a lot of friends as a kid though. Isn't that usually the way it goes? Lots of friends as a kid and then as you grow they fall by the wayside and by the time you hit thirty you're lucky if you have five true friends? At least, there's some saying that goes something like that, about when you die. I did have a bunch though. Rachel was one of my best friends for a time because our dads worked together. She lived at the back of my neighborhood and we would climb the wall and go to the liquor store that used to be called The Cracker Barrel, but I think it's since changed its name. I got my first sting by a wasp in her front yard when I leaned up against a tree with a wasp just chillin right beneath where I put my hand. This, logically, taught me to always look where I was putting my hands.

Another very good friend of mine was the previously mentioned Courtney. Her family moved to Buffalo, New York in the fifth grade and I never saw her again. I remember one evening when my mother had been on the phone for what felt like ages and I wanted to ask her if Courtney could come over so I made a sign that simply said "can Courtney come over?" but she didn't respond to my sign. I don't know how I would have called Courtney to see if she was available because this was well before the internet and cell phones and we had only one landline, which my mother was occupying. In any case, somehow that I don't remember, I broke a glass on the kitchen floor, and I meant to clean it up, but something distracted me and I didn't, and my mother cut her foot on it. I often wonder if somehow, subconsciously, I wanted my mother to cut her foot for ignoring me. I was only about six and I really don't think I would have wanted that to happen. I wish I could say this is where I learned to clean up my messes and finish what I'm doing before started something else, but I've always been easily distracted, and it's only gotten worse with time.

I was definitely a creative child. I had an easel in the basement and loved to paint and draw. I would finger paint and use brushes to make all kinds of pictures, many of which I still have to this day in my giant yellow Crayola portfolio with the rest of my more recent work. As I got older, I really grew into designing spaces. I moved bedrooms in my house just so I could redesign my room from scratch. I painted each wall a different, vibrant color, and put my bed in the closet, which was just barely big enough for a twin mattress, but not a box spring or frame. This lasted for a few years, but then I moved back to my original room which I redecorated one summer with light blue cloud wall paper, a pink glittery ceiling, (I threw glitter up in small doses onto areas I had coated with spray adhesive and I do NOT recommend this method) and a pink rug with a homemade bed cut to resemble a cloud underneath my rainbow bedspread. I even painted the Lisa Frank unicorns on my closet doors. I thought it was just magical. My dad helped quite a bit with this one.

The summer before second grade I even starred in and directed a play based on Aladdin, which was a live action movie, before Disney released their animated version. Courtney was a dancer and had all these fancy costumes from frequent recitals that were rather universally sized for kids our age, and I casted her as the genie, a couple boys from our class as the Sultan and Aladdin, and I, of course, was Princess Jasmine. My dad helped build some pretty mediocre scenery. Nothing against his craftsmanship, he was a carpenter's apprentice for some time, so he knew what he was doing, but looking back, my paintings that hung from the wood frames of fabulous temples and palaces in fluorescent tempura paints weren't exactly my personal best work. We even had a "magic lamp" which I'm pretty sure was actually a gravy boat. We held several rehearsals, and made flyers, and all of our families came to my house to watch my little play. I didn't even realize what a task this all was for a seven year old. My dad told me much later in life that all the kids in the neighborhood always looked up to me, and if there was ever an issue that needed solving, they'd all look to me for the answer. These are likely idealized memories from a doting father.

I also remember around first grade going to a store with my mother, and there was this little set of pink and purple heart-shaped erasers that I wanted. She told me I couldn't get them, so I stole them and hid them under a hat on the dresser in my room. This was apparently not a good hiding place as she found them a day or two later and told me she was taking me back to the store so I could return them to the owner and apologize. This never happened though. I think she was too embarrassed because she just ran into the store and put them back on the shelf. I believe this is what initially taught me that it is okay to steal, as long as you don't get caught.

We belonged to a swim club for a few years when I was younger. My mother thought it was the cat's meow and went all the time. My dad's visits were far less often, but I do remember one particular day when he came along and I could tell they were fighting, as usual. I sat on the bench with my dad facing the playground eating our ice cream cones and I asked him, in my best seven-year-old-too-wise-for-my-years-voice: "Daddy? How long are you and Mommy gonna stay married?" And he responded that he was going to stay married to my mother as long as he could. It was that very night that my younger brother, Tom, and I were awoken in the middle of the night to my mother screaming up the stairs that they were getting a divorce.

Tom and I were given the choice which parent we wanted to live with to avoid messy custody battles and Tom chose to stay with my dad and I chose to go with my mother. In these days, I thought my mother needed my protection. We were going to be best friends and go shopping and have girl time and it was going to be great! This is not what happened. She was determined to find someone and remarry before my father (who wasn't even looking) and was in every club and choir she could be a part of. I would go to school, stay after in "latchkey" with the other kids whose parents worked, (like my new friends Aaron and Rob,) my dad would come get us around six, we'd go home to his house, and then my mother would come get me around ten, or whenever she was done doing whatever it was that she was doing. It went on like this for months.

     The other issue was, how shall I put this delicately...my mother was in no mental state to be caring for a child at this time. Let's just say my mother had a pretty crappy childhood. I know lots of people think they had it bad, but she really did for reasons I will not get into. She suppressed a lot of it, but the trauma of the divorce brought it all back up, and basically, she lost it, for lack of a more medically accurate term. She spent some time in the mental ward of the hospital where I was born, and when she came home, I remember several instances of her freaking out uncontrollably for no apparent reason. One night she was sitting on the edge of her bed in her nightgown rocking back and forth while clutching her creamsicle-colored stuffed hippo she had named "hugs," crying and calling me "mommy." I was eight.

More Than Real*2002

Sometimes a child cries out for water
In the middle of the night
But mommy and sister, they didn't cry for water
They fought back not thirst, but fright

For sister cried out for water once
Had a glass of it poured on her head
Now forced to sleep in wet pajamas
Fighting back tears instead

And sometimes you tell no one
How daddy makes you feel
And sometimes those monsters under the bed
Are a little more than real

Sometimes a child awakens
From nightmarish sleep, in screams
But for mommy, waking was the nightmare
She was safe within her dreams

And sometimes she still awakens
And cries out, out of fright
But she awakens not for thirst of dreams
But the memory of those nights

And sometimes you tell no one
How daddy makes you feel
And sometimes those monsters under the bed
Are a little more than real

~*~

I begged her to let me go back to living with my father, but she refused. I don't remember her reasons, whatever they were. My father was paying her child support on top of what he had already paid her in the divorce settlement, which was substantial, and he was also paying her an additional several hundred dollars per month to stay in the Birmingham School District, because they were the best in the area. Top three in the country, or so I heard at one point. It wasn't until he agreed to continue paying her this child support money, in the form of alimony, that she agreed to let me move back home with my dad, but I'm sure she'll deny that. Frankly, I would.

My brother and I continued to visit her every other weekend. She dated here and there and usually had a new man every year or few. I generally didn't like them, but let's be fair, what young girl is going to like her mother's new boyfriends when she loves her dad so much, which I did. I remember one of them was apparently pretty wealthy and had very bad teeth. He bought her a real fur coat and took us up in his little Cessna airplane. My mother liked that he would call from his car phone when he would arrive because she hated the sound of the buzzer to her apartment. It's funny the things we remember, isn't it?

The one I remember the most was Rob. He was twenty-three when my mother met him at some nudist singles weekend thing and they started dating. I was twelve. She was turning forty that year. Funny small-world story here: he was still living with his mother, Tamara, whom, as we discovered later, my dad had a crush on when they went to high school together! Yes, I'll allow you a minute to process that one. My mother was now dating the son of a woman my dad had gone to school with. Yes, very weird for me. He was really much more like my older brother. He looked quite a bit like Kurt Cobain, as really any man with long dirty blonde hair did in those days, especially after not shaving for a few days, which Rob didn't really do very often.

One year, he took us to the Rainbow Gathering, which, if you're unfamiliar with, is basically a big hippie fest in some remote area that moves around the country and clothing is optional. I think I was thirteen by this point, my brother would have been eleven, and of course, we wore clothing, as did my mother only because we were present, but Rob did not. I didn't really understand how the food and water worked and didn't eat or drink anything for almost 3 days, and needless to say was extremely dehydrated upon return, and couldn't even get out of bed the next morning without passing out.

Rob wanted me to call him "dad," which I refused to do. I had a father and he wasn't it. And he was only ten years older than me, it wasn't even possible. But, one day, when my mother and Rob were moving into a house they had just bought together, I used my powers of female manipulation, called him "dad," and got him to let me and my friends ride in the back of the empty moving truck on a trip back to the apartment, on rollerblades. Fortunately, for us, this is where that story ends. I realize for the sake of this book it would be a lot more interesting if someone had actually broken a limb or we'd gotten into some horrible accident, but no, everyone did, I'm sorry to say, survive.

Rob was also the enabler to my getting drunk the first time. My friend, Emily, was supposed to be staying over, and she asked him to buy us beer and wine; and then of course, her parents changed their mind once they learned that Rob would be there and she had to go home, so Rob had this beer and wine for just me. We waited for my mother to go to bed, and then he taught me drinking games like bounce the quarter into the shoe, and likely several others, but I don't remember much about that night aside from getting violently ill, and him waking me up in a closet I had either just sat down in, or passed out in, and putting me into my bed. I was soaking wet all over, I assume from trying to sweat out the alcohol. My mother woke in the night to the sound of my throwing up and just assumed I was sick, and so she called me into school the next day, thank goodness. I honestly don't think I was this sick for another seventeen years. This, is why I didn't drink again for a very long time.

Eventually my mother tired of taking care of essentially a third child and asked him to move out. She had a few roommates here and there, but I don't remember any of them staying too long. She was somewhat difficult to live with. One particular weekend she had gone grocery shopping at the local Food Lion, as it was called at the time. Upon her exit from the store she was walking to her car, with her purse in the cart and a car pulled up beside her and a man got out, flashed a gun and said "this is an armed robbery." For some reason, my mother grabbed her purse out of the cart as if to hold it closer, but the man snatched it from her, jumped back into the car, and they sped away. She started yelling, someone called the police, and they were caught all of five minutes later I believe, but the police needed to hold on to her things for a few days for evidence. This was Saturday. On her way to the police station on Tuesday to pick up her belongings, she got into a pretty bad car accident that totaled her car; but she walked away bruised but nothing broken. She believes this is because there was a bible in the trunk of her car.

She was always into the church before, but never like she was after that car wreck. She started going to church several times a week, and quoting scripture left and right, and "cleansing" her household waving sticks of burning sage, I think, around from room to room. My brother was very into Anime, and she wouldn't let him watch Pokémon, one of his favorite shows at the time because in her eyes it was "violent." I was also feeling sick one weekend at her place, and was watching one of my favorite movies, *The Princess Bride*, and she walked in right when Indigo Montoya is about to avenge his father's death and she told me to turn it off because it was too violent, and somehow I managed to convince her that it was justice he was fighting for. This only worked for about a minute though because she came back in claiming that no, it was vengeance, and that was a sin and she wouldn't have sin in her house. So, fortunately for Tom and myself, I had a car by this point, had recently earned my driver's license, ironically thanks to her, and we packed up our things and went back home to dad's house. I don't know if Tom went over to her house again, honestly. I saw her here and there for about the next year because I had a car, and I've always believed in the inherent good in people, and like it or not, she was still my mother.

That fall I took an English electives class about great works of literature that have drastically influenced cultures, and we spent the first third of the semester talking about different stories in the bible. One particular section I had to write a paper about was the story of Abraham and Isaac. For those who are not familiar with the story: God tests Abraham and asks him to sacrifice his only beloved son. When God sees that Abraham has every intention of doing so, an angel swoops in, basically tells him "just kidding," and shows him a ram in the thicket to sacrifice instead. What I could not wrap my mind around was the concept of sacrificing your own child. I realized, however, that I didn't have the faith that Abraham must've had. Hell, I was practically an atheist at this point in my life, so I called my mother.

I explained what I was studying and what the paper was about and asked her if God told her to kill me if she would. Her response was "well, I hope this doesn't upset you, but the bible tells us to love God first, then ourselves, and then our families, so yes, if God told me to kill you, then I would trust he had a plan and I would have to kill you." I slept on the floor of my room for the next week as opposed to the bed which was up against the window. I had recently learned that the theory on dreams is that they are your short term memories being transferred to your long term memory, and I was convinced having this conversation was going to cause her to have a dream where God told her to kill me, and she would think that was actually him talking to her. This was twelve years ago though and I'm still alive, thank God.

At the end of the summer after my senior year of high school, after I turned eighteen and my dad didn't have to keep paying her ridiculous sums of money every month for nothing, she realized she couldn't afford to support herself on her secretarial job and decided to move back in with her parents in Savannah, Georgia. She sold her house, which you could actually do in those days, took her small profit with her, and I helped with the driving. Actually, I think I did all the driving because I hated the way that she drove. She was so bent on following rules that she wouldn't go one mile an hour over the limit, so as opposed to just maintaining speed just under or even at the limit, she would accelerate until she hit the limit, then take her foot off the gas pedal, then re-accelerate until she was just at the limit again; it was nauseating. Savannah was beautiful though. It is my favorite city in this country and I have often said if my mother didn't live there, I would. Cobblestone streets, little shops right along the river downtown, and Spanish moss draped over everything. Just, charming.

She went to Mustard Seed Seminary School for a few years and earned an associates in seminary studies. I didn't talk to her as much as I probably should have for a little while, but what did I really have to say. She was "married to Jesus" now and I was a college student in the throes of my youth and experimentation days, so anything I would have had to talk about probably would have been met with further suggestions to turn to Jesus. Which, especially in those days, I was not inclined to do. She eventually went to Armstrong Atlantic State University and graduated with a Bachelors in Liberal Arts. She has had several administrative positions since.

CHAPTER 2

Well, now that you've met my mother, let me introduce you to my dad. He was pretty awesome. A pretty free spirit who never took anything too seriously, but the few things in life that mattered to him most. He was a self-proclaimed fat kid that lost all the weight in high-school, was popular enough to be known around a campus of 45,000 students at Michigan State, where he went for almost ten years without graduating. He spent years traveling about the country from the beaches of Fort Lauderdale, to Pasadena for the Rose Bowl one year, even though State lost, and had all kinds of odd jobs. It wasn't until he checked himself into a mental institution because he thought something might be wrong with him, and some guy in a group said "you're smart, you should go into computers" that he found his life's calling. Now, realize, this was in the early seventies when a single computer still took up half a room, and computers were a new technology; but my dad had always been interested in science and math, and tinkering with gadgets and whatnot. He got a night job as a security guard so he could do his homework, and put himself through Oakland Community College during the day. I imagine there were some jobs in between, but at some early point, he hooked up with Pete Karmanos, and helped him build Compuware, now one of the nation's leading software corporations; out of a building no bigger than the A&W it was next to with maybe twelve guys. He was very proud of being smart.

Now, I'm not saying he was the greatest father. After the divorce the first thing he taught us children was how to do our own laundry so he wouldn't have to. The first thing he bought was a microwave, because he was not about to start cooking meals. Every night it was "what do you kids want for dinner? McDonald's? Burger King? Wendy's?" There was always food in the house, but he let us pick what we wanted, so it was Coke and chips, not milk and vegetables. He walked in on his own surprise party when he was younger, so he hated surprises. He would take us to the toy store before Christmas and let us pick out what we wanted and then we'd come home and I'd wrap everything, because boy do I love wrapping presents. (For real, I was even a professional gift wrapper one season at a local toy store. Love it.) He always let us do whatever we wanted, within reason, but it was rare we wanted to do anything out of reason, so as long as he knew where we would be and when we'd be home, we were allowed to go. But there was a respect level there and I never pushed the rules, so I don't know what the punishment would have been had I come home late. I imagine I would not have been allowed to go to the next thing.

He liked buying us things. I remember one weekend coming home from my mother's to a new trampoline in the backyard. I loved that thing. I had my tenth birthday party out there in bathing suits, while it was raining and probably fifty degrees. He also let us know he would help buy our first car. Whatever we saved, he would match that amount. He would also cover the insurance for the first year (which I think turned into four years for me) and he would put new brakes on it, if it needed them. I got a bright yellow 1994 Geo Tracker with a black soft top that came off in pieces, and boy did I love that car. I still mourn that car. My friends called it the S.U.wannaV. I made tie-dyed seat covers for it, glued quarters to the dashboard in honor of my movie boyfriend, A.J., put stickers all over it, and it was the best representation of my personality in that time, as I was always wearing the brightest, loudest clothes I could find, and had at least seven different colors in my hair at a given time. We got searched every single time we crossed the border to Canada, but they never found anything because even though we certainly looked like pot smoking hippies, none of us had ever touched the stuff. We were the choir nerds. But I'm getting off topic.

Bottom line: my dad was pretty sweet. I remember coming home from school one day after he had left Compuware, and there was a note on our whiteboard in the entry hallway that simply read:

"Kids, gone to the beach. −dad"

which my friend, Elena, thought was hysterical. I'm guessing she never came home to such notes, but this was common in my house. He taught me everything I needed to know without my even knowing how he was teaching me. I didn't know until many years later that he actually made decent money, but he taught me how to work if I wanted something. He believed you need a college degree to get anywhere in this world, and made me go to college, and stay in college when I begged to drop out midway through my freshman year. He would not replace things if they were broken or lost, we had to save up our own money and buy it again. He gave us pretty extensive chores because frankly, he didn't want to clean or cut the grass or really do much around the house, but we were compensated fairly.

He sent me off to summer camp for just a week when I was maybe eight or so and I loved it. I went back year after year for two weeks and then three. I made so many friends and had such a good time; it was my favorite place to be in the world and I wept like a baby at the end of every session. By the summer before high school I loved it so much I wanted to go for an extra two weeks the next summer, but my dad was only willing to pay for the four he'd already committed to. So, the second semester of my freshman year, I got a babysitting job about a mile from my school and I walked there every day after school to take care of the kid and saved up the money to pay for another two weeks of summer camp. I'm sure my dad could have afforded it, but he didn't want me to become a spoiled brat, and now, I really appreciate that and would have done the same.

We used to have these talks every so often, maybe only twice a year. Later into the night, if I couldn't sleep, I would come down the stairs, and there he would be, in his chair, in the family room in front of our TV and computer in one that he made before that sort of thing even existed and we would just talk about who knows what. I can't even give you an example, but looking back, those are some of my favorite moments. I'm sure whatever he was working on was really important to him, but as soon as I'd walk in, he'd put it on hold.

I didn't handle my teenage years well. I mean, honestly, who does, right? I could have been much worse, but I also could have been much better. My dad had studied psychology for a time at Michigan State, so he used to constantly tell me all these thoughts and emotions and phases as a teenager I "should" go through. I hated that. I remember saying "you don't understand" to him, only once, and he got this look on his face like he was such a proud father because I'd officially become a teenager, and I huffed and ran upstairs to my room, but then didn't even slam the door like I was going to because this would have only proven him right, that I was being a typical teenager.

When I was about thirteen, some plans I had with some of my summer camp friends fell through. I knew a lot of the counselors were still at the camp staying year round because school groups would come every weekend and they needed a skeleton crew to do activities with the kids. I knew that my counselor, Sandi, who I had idealized and turned into my second mother in my mind, was there. So, I walked. It was about an hour away by car and I did the math as I was walking that I could make it by morning and not have to get in anyone's car, but by the time I made it to the freeway, a nice man pulled over and offered me a ride, so I accepted. He was actually kind of cute, very nice, probably early twenties, no idea what his name was, but he took me to my exit. I lied about him though because I knew everyone would worry he tried to rape me or something, so I said he was a she, her name was Rachel, she was 23 and had long blonde hair. When I got to the top of my exit I looked in either direction as far as I could see and honestly didn't know which way it was. It seemed so simple when my dad drove me, but I didn't remember whether we turned left or right, and it was dark; and yes, logic and geography now tells me that it would have had to be right because Holly is very north of 96, but I didn't think like this when I was only thirteen. I even went into the gas station to ask directions, but they had no idea what I was talking about. So I guessed, and thankfully, I made the right choice, and started walking north.

The grass on the side of the road was very tall and very wet, and there was no sidewalk. I hadn't told anyone where I was going, just "for a walk," so I'm sure everyone back home was worried sick, but again, this was still before cell phones. Thank God some nice old men, a pair of them, pulled over to see if I needed help and drove me the rest of the way to where I was going, which ended up being easily another ten miles or more up the road. When I got there, I went straight to the lodge where I knew the counselors generally stayed and found out from the one there that Sandi was out, but he made me call my dad and tell him where I was. He, obviously, told me to stay put, he was coming to get me right away and no, I absolutely could not stay the night. It took him about forty five minutes to get there and I got to see Sandi for a little while, but I think I scared her something fierce, this 13 year old girl just showing up at probably ten at night, crying about how no one is keeping in touch from the summer. She didn't come back the next year, and I think she only wrote to me one more time. My dad didn't say anything on the way home. He was clearly terrified, but relieved. I think he felt partially responsible, but I don't know why. It only came up once or twice, that terrible night that I walked up to camp. I don't even think I was punished for what I'd done, but I could see it in his face that I'd taken years off his life that night. This is the last time I went anywhere without telling him where I was going.

I also had a very bad episode involving a bunch of sleeping pills and a night in the hospital which I imagine cost him an exorbitant amount of money because we didn't have health insurance at the time, but I've already apologized to him about that, profusely. I was seventeen and it was the first time in a year or more that my high school sweetheart and I were not going to see each other that day, and we were having problems. I was so dreadfully "in love" with him that I thought this was the end of the world, but fortunately, it was not. I got over it, we broke up, he started seeing my best friend behind by back not too long after, and everyone hid it from me until I figured it out and the world ended all over again. High school drama. Gross. At least this heartache caused my dad to agree to pay for the Florida Keys spring break trip through the school I wanted to go on that he originally said no to. This was how he fixed things. Just buy something until it's all better.

Lovers' Hell*2002

When was my demotion
From the twinkle in your eye
When came my replacement
As the sun in your sky
When came the day
That your eyes turned to grey
Why am I no longer your prize

Now that you've conquered
And shackled this heart
You leave me no option
When the thunder starts
No matter the lightening
Or the rains pouring so hard
My chains won't let me flee the dark

Send me back to lovers' hell
It's a place I've come to know so well
Love is just a game
That I will never learn to play
Send me back to lovers' hell

When was I removed from
That corner in your mind
The one that you retreat to
In the worst of times
I don't know what happened
If the fault is really mine
I don't remember refusing to shine

No, I am still that princess
You met not long ago
The one that you slew dragons for
The one that you loved so
What happened to the fires
That I used to know
Where did your love
For me go

Send me back to lovers' hell
It's a place I've come to know so well
Their armors rusted through
I should have known that yours would too
Send me back to lovers' hell

Send me back to lovers' hell

It's a place I've come to know so well
If you never play the game
Then it never ends in pain
Send me back to lovers' hell

I'm going home to lovers' hell
It's a place I've come to know oh so well
I'm turning in my keys
Hope has given up on me
I'm going home to lovers' hell

Yeah I'm going home to lovers' hell
But I've made my home in love…

~*~

I also went through a brief phase in my teen years when I discovered I could belch incredibly loudly when I wanted to after drinking carbonated beverages. He always used to say to me in his scolding tone: "Jenniferrrrrr….nobody loves a farting princess." To which I would respond that I had burped, not farted, but he said it was generally the same thing. It was basically his way of telling me that it was very un-lady-like. I swear he told me once what that phrase was from, some book or movie or something, but I don't remember. I've asked everyone I know and googled the piss out of it, but can't find it. Do you know? If you do know, please contact me. It's probably copyrighted material and I'm going to get sued. That will be fun.

He was also one of the funniest people I ever knew, but maybe that's just because he was my dad. One of my favorite stories about him is a time we were walking our dog, Oreo, and somehow it came up what we wanted done with our remains when we passed. I said some hippie crap about wanting my ashes tossed in an easterly wind at sunrise over the ocean or something. He, after a brief pause said he'd like to be bronzed and turned into a lamp so that he could live forever going from garage sale to garage sale. I laughed so hard I nearly wet myself.

CHAPTER 3

So, you know that I was a creative child, I didn't handle my teenage years well, and you've met my mother and father. If you're wondering about my brother, we don't really have much of a relationship. Aside from our early years where we bickered as much as any other young siblings do, we've never really had much in common. He likes video games and Japanese animation, and staying inside and keeping all of his friends online, where as I always have to be doing something and until recently, didn't do much sitting still. My mother has a favorite story where I wrote his name on the wall as a child trying to get him in trouble, overlooking the fact he was barely capable of even holding a crayon at that point in time. We get along just fine and promised my dad we'd call each other on their birthday, but beyond that, we never know what to say. He never went to camp, or really left the house as a kid much. I, personally taught him how to ride a bike around the age of sixteen or so because my dad paid us each a hundred bucks. He never learned to drive a car, but he's gotten pretty good at the various bus systems in the random cities he's lived in. He has a bachelor's degree in Economics from Wayne State University, has since earned another bachelor's in Accounting from Ashford University, and is currently working towards a master's degree in Computer Sciences, from Armstrong Atlantic State University, in Savannah, Georgia, where my mother went. He only recently acquired his first "real" job. He bussed tables and did dishes at a couple restaurants, but they both closed, and I don't even think he got paid for one of them because they hired him all of two weeks before they closed, so I'm sure they knew they were going to be closing. He's very smart, but rather lacking in social graces.

Um, where was I? Well, let's pick up around the end of high school as I think we've covered all the relevant material up to this point. I was the social chairman of the choir for three years straight, (freshmen couldn't run because they're chosen the year before) uncontested for two of them. I planned parties, and lock-ins and picnics and all kinds of fun things. I was also a lead in the spring musical three years running; Hodel in Fiddler on the Roof, Irene Malloy in Hello Dolly and Audrey in Little Shop of Horrors. I didn't audition freshmen year because I was babysitting, but you knew that already. I really enjoyed the stage, particularly singing. I wrote a song for my graduation which I was honored to perform in front of a few thousand people at our commencement ceremony, which is also one of the highlights of my life. My friend, Elena, and I made fairy wings that we wore during the procession; prompting a new rule for following ceremonies that nothing could be worn outside the gown. I also designed and sewed my own prom dress inspired by the nymph character in one of my brother's Dungeons and Dragons books. It was sea-foam green with ripped-looking edges, rope straps and wrapped around my torso, and I had ivy running up my leg with flowers in my hair. It earned me a centerfold in the senior edition of the yearbook. A picture of it is also in my art portfolio.

It was also during my senior year that somehow, my friends and I discovered that Canada was only twenty minutes away, and they had veggie burgers at their McDonald's, and they didn't ID for tattoos and piercings, and just had way cooler things to buy at their mall, for way cheaper because the exchange rate was way better in those days. I usually drove, and like I mentioned earlier, we literally got searched every time we went over. You didn't even need a passport in those days, a photo ID and birth certificate would suffice. In March or April, one of my best friends, Leah, and I decided to get tattoos. She got a pretty swirly blue flash piece on her hip. I wanted fairy wings on my back, but ended up with the trashiest set of rainbow colored butterfly-looking cartoon wings that three hundred American dollars could buy. I was proud of them for about a month until the seventy first person said "cool butterfly." I just stopped correcting people. There was a separate piercing place called "Need a New Hole" and I got just about everything pierced that I could hide from my dad. He had let me get my navel done when I was thirteen, and then my eyebrow, which he wasn't happy about. I had two hundred of my schoolmates sign a petition freshman year that tongue rings were cool, so he finally agreed to that but made me promise no more. I didn't keep that promise very long. By my eighteenth birthday I had seven holes in each ear, both eyebrows, my tongue, my navel, both nipples and clit hood; the last three of which my dad did not know about. Shortly thereafter I got my septum done which I could flip up inside my nose, and did my own lip, which dad made me take out, but I re-pierced it a few years later, along with my nostril.

The year I graduated, my drama teacher started a summer troupe of alumni and started putting on a play every year, the first of which was The Rimers of Eldridge. It was a rather unconventional play that bounced around a lot, had the whole cast on the stage the entire time, had no scenes, only jumped from one section to another for two acts, but I loved it. I was initially cast in a small role, but when the girl's parents read the script for the role that I wanted, Eva, they pulled her out and I got it. Eva is a young girl, probably twelve or so and she's slightly disfigured, walks with a limp. She's an only child with a very over-protective single mother and is very naïve. I loved her innocence. She has a good friend who is a boy nearly six years her senior and he snaps near the end of the play and tries to rape her in the woods. She screams and the neighborhood crazy homeless man intervenes, saving her, but another neighbor overhears, runs to the scene and mistakenly shoots the homeless man and kills him, and Eva can't say anything because she's too terrified, so everything just goes back to the way it was before. This was the most fun I ever had on a play, even though there was no music in it. I loved all the new people I had met; Steve, in particular. We started dating right before I left for college. He had very pretty eyes, and could cry on command, which I'm sure he used on me at least once or twice. We had a good six months before it all went to hell and I never heard from him again, likely for the better.

My Sailor*2002

I was standing on the pier
Waiting for my sailor
To take me away from here
And show me love that's true
I was frightened of that water
And everything unclear
But as the sun was rising
His sails came in view

With eyes that shined like silver
Skin warmer than the sand
Kissed me so gently
And took my hand
Said please my frightened angel
I'll show you worlds you've only dreamed
But you must leave your shoreline
Come away with me

Tell me you'll wait
And simply understand

That I nearly drowned
The last time I left the sand

I said my love, I'm sorry
I'm just not set to said
He said my love, just have faith
Love will always prevail
But he started getting restless
Giving up on me
And as the sun was setting
He left me for the sea

Darling, why leave me
Did you not know?
I was well over waist deep
Nearly set to go
I'd battled all my demons
Swallowed all my pride
It took everything inside me
To step into the tide

Cuz you said you'd wait
Said you'd understand
But you didn't wait
Now I'm crying in the sand

And now I'm standing on the pier
Longing for my sailor
Who left me crying here
The way I knew he'd do
All the more frightened of that water
And everything unclear
For although the sun keeps rising
Love just isn't true

For you said you'd wait
Til I was set to go
But you didn't wait

Well my love,
I told you so

~*~

That summer, I also met Jack, who honestly, I thought was out of my league. He was a few years older, had dreadlocks and a lip ring, and I was so turned on by him, that he intimidated me. I don't even know why, honestly. I had already given my virginity to my high school sweetheart. Well, to be honest, I offered it, he didn't even ask, but we were going to be together forever and get married anyway, so I figured why wait? Right? Yeah. So, I hadn't been pure for almost two years, but, I had never been turned on the way I was around him, and he liked me! But for some reason, I was so, I don't know, nervous, overwhelmed, by how much I wanted him that I didn't call him back, even after he called me to hang out, a few times.

Sleeping with El Sol*2001
(Spoken word piece)

The sun is beginning to awaken
But I have yet to sleep.
Peeking over the horizon,
Lighting my humble room and me on my computer
Debating with the idea of crawling into the bed.
Not particularly sleepy, but feeling rather obligated to rest.
My body treats me well, and I suppose I should return the favor.
Recharge my battery before beginning a new day.

So much left to do.
Sleeping seems such a waste of time.

But if I sleep, perhaps I'll have a moment's freedom from the thoughts of you that plague me. Haven't seen you in 4 days, probably won't for several more, than not for weeks after that, if ever again.

We agreed to keep it casual, I warned you of my fear. Said I'd run screaming if I started to fall, but now I'm falling and screaming but not running, and apparently not sleeping and only thinking, thinking about you and your lovely little way of cleverly agreeing to the terms of our casual "not relationship" and then twisting the rules right out from under me. Didn't make me come to you, but backed me up to the edge and let me fall. You're winning, I'm falling, I'm screaming, was doing so well, now it all goes to hell since you kissed me.

My lips may not have been upon yours since that day but I haven't stopped kissing you. For three hours they never parted, for 4 days they've still felt you. Do I run, do I stay, do I fall, do I pull you down with me? Do I go to sleep because tomorrow I am one day closer to saying goodbye? Do I stay awake because I don't know that goodbye is what I want for I was sure that I wouldn't fall but I did but I can still be saved. In three weeks I move away. There is time only for several more visits between now and then anyhow. Perhaps if I loved you for just a few hours.

No.

I will not fall in love.

Perhaps if we kiss for just a few hours more, but do not fall in love.

If we giggle and play but then move away, and see others as though nothing had happened.
I won't fall, I won't run, I won't scream...

I won't love.

However, I think I will sleep.

The sun thinks I should sleep.

~*~

Jack and his friends however, were "freegans." They only ate what they could get for free (most of the time). Sometimes this meant dumpster diving, and sometimes this meant shoplifting. Remember when I mentioned I never learned stealing was bad as a child? Even though I only saw Jack a few times, I started shoplifting, and I got good at it.

There were rules though. Rule number one: always buy something. Don't ever walk out of the store with stolen goods without making a purchase. Rule number two: only from big, evil corporations that probably have a "theft budget" line on their Profit and Loss statements. Rule number three: never get too comfortable. Once you stop paying attention, you get caught. I even made a large purse with easy openings specifically for shoplifting. I could slip just about anything in there. My personal best was a pair of boots I really wanted, from a smaller shop that certainly broke rule number two. They were a foot high heel and they went more than halfway up the calf, so they were no small feat (no pun intended). I managed to slip one into my shoplifting bag but knowing the other wouldn't fit I called to my friend across the store that I was going to put money in the meter and would be right back. I did put money in the meter, but I also put the boot in my car, and went back and snagged the other one. I'm not proud of it now, but I can't lie, I sure was that day. Leah, who was also in on this bad habit took a choker right off a mannequin. We were so proud of ourselves. We'll come back to this though.

Being that my dad loved Michigan State so much, I think it was just assumed I would go there. I applied to a total of four schools, and got into all of them, but I ultimately ended up going to Michigan State. One trip up to see the campus was all I needed. The trees were amazing. I never even went to the other three. My dad couldn't be happier. The only problem was, Steve was staying home in the Southfield area and commuting to Wayne State; and most of my friends were a year younger and in their senior year of high school, back home, except Leah, who was also going to Wayne State. I didn't know anyone at Michigan State and despite how social I was in high school, I was not very good at meeting people I didn't already know, unlike my father. I went home every weekend, except for the one that Steve and I drove out to Chicago to get my tattoo covered by James Kern, a renowned inksmith that I had discovered in a tattoo magazine clipping on the wall in the bathroom of the local tattoo studio on campus. That did not cost three hundred dollars. He charged $175 an hour in those days and he worked on me about eight hours over two days. A few years later I had them added onto when he was in town for the Motor City Tattoo Expo and his rate had gone up to $200 an hour and he worked on me for another ten hours, and then four more hours the next year. You can do the math. To this day, I have no idea where that money came from. The quality of the work was completely worth it however, and I will never go to another artist. It's so faded at this point, but I don't have the money to fly out to Portland, where he is now. Or the money to get it touched up to begin with.

I do think there was one key factor that may have helped me learn to like State. I auditioned for one of their A Cappella groups called Capital Green as I had been big into choir and our A Cappella group in high school. I almost made it. I even got a call-back. But alas, the poor fellow who called to let me know the director wanted the other girl swore he would have chosen me, but it was not his choice to make. He was probably just being nice. I cried, but I'm a big crybaby. You'll come to learn this about me. I do think had I made it into that group I would have immediately gained a group of friends that already went to the school and could show me around and take me to parties and introduce me to the Spartan lifestyle. However, I did not, so I went home every weekend and hung out with Steve and my creative friends that all went to Wayne State, where I should have gone in the first place. Around December Leah introduced me to some new people she'd just met in her apartment building on Prentis Street in midtown Detroit, and my life, quite literally, changed forever.

CHAPTER 4

I believe it was the week between Christmas and New Years and I was home on break for a bit. Leah was incredibly musically gifted and was going to Wayne State for music, I believe. She called me one day and told me about this open-mic night I had to come to because she wanted me to meet her new friend, Blair, who was teaching her to play the guitar. He hosted it every Sunday night at a café in Ferndale I'd been to a few times, called Xhedo's. I was enthralled. There were poets and singer/songwriters and everyone who signed up could do three pieces or fifteen minutes, whichever came first. Blair, as the host, would insert a song or a poem here or there before introducing the next act. I also met his roommate, Dale Wilson, and another musician, Dan Minard, and another open-mic host, Sean Fitzgerald. They were all very talented musicians. Leah, apparently hit the jackpot of budding artists by moving into this particular building, with our other gifted friend, Sally, to attend Wayne State. I have to admit, I was a bit jealous. Over the next few months I taught myself to play the guitar (very poorly), wrote a few songs, and even got up on stage and performed a few times, at Blair's request, under the stage name "Pixie," which many of those people still call me. I was terrible, but Blair had this way of making you think you were better than you were and that every performance is just experience for the next one. He made you want to get better.

Mirror Mirror*2002

Night after night 'til the first signs of light
I try and I try with all of my might
I practice for hours, to no avail
No matter how I hard I try, I still seem to fail
I have to keep going, my head towards the sky
But when I when I seem to get nowhere, it's so hard to try

I want to be good like you
I want to be talented too
I want to play the way that you do
I want to be loved like you

I want to feel that rush from the crowd
Simply for pouring my heart out
Though it remains to be seen who I'm trying to please
When the sound of my voice brings a man to his knees
Maybe then I'll be satisfied

But what if that day never comes...

I've got a devil on one shoulder, the other is bare
I'm my own worst critic, my own worst nightmare
That mirror mirror on the wall
Saying "you'll never make it to the best of them all
"So why don't you finally admit you're defeat
"No matter how hard you try, you'll never join the elite"

I want to be good like you
I want to be talented too
I want to play the way that you do
I want to be loved like you

I want to feel the rush from the crowd
Simply for pouring my heart out
Though I've tried and I've tried, through all of the years

When the sound of my voice brings a grown man to tears
Maybe then I'll be satisfied

But what if that day never comes
What if that day never comes
What if that day...

~*~

I remember keeping a journal during this time and I would
write down nice or funny things that people would say and I
remember it said "Dan Minard said HE would OPEN for ME
when I start playing shows!" I was like a teeny-bopper for these
people; it was pretty ridiculous. They were just all so good.
Blair, Dale, Sean, and Dan, as well as Marcus, Audra, Ian, Tone
and Niche, Allison Lewis, Hugo, and Lisa Hurt were some of my
favorites. There were many others, but we'd be here for days if
I mentioned every open-mic-er that I was enthralled with.
There was one that I was particularly enthralled with, and I'm
pretty sure the entire state of Michigan knew I was enthralled
with him. Let me tell you, there is no greater confidence
booster than attaining someone you really want, but thought
you would never have. Even if it's only for one drunken, blurry
night.

Unrequited*2002

I'm sorry her beautiful face
Isn't the one that I wear
I'm sorry her beautiful name
Isn't the one that I bare
I'm sorry that I'm not enough
I'm sorry I can't ease your pain
I'm trying to warm your heart
I guess I'll just love you in vain

She wants what she can't have
Can't see what she's got
But I'm the one who loves you
While she loves you not
I know when you hold me
You're thinking of her
But yours are the only
Arms I prefer

I'm sorry I don't have the power
To bring back her feelings for you
All I want is for you to be happy
But it seems that there's nothing I can do

I'm sorry I won't feed you lies
And I'm sorry I won't waste your time
I'm so sorry her beautiful eyes
Can't see you the way that do mine

She wants what she can't have
Can't see what she's got
But I'm the one who loves you
While she loves you not
And I know when you hold me
You wish I was her
But yours are the only
Arms I prefer

Maybe if I didn't love you
If I could just walk away
Maybe then you'd notice
Finally want me to stay
I know why you're crying
I feel the same way for you
If you can't be with the one you love
No one else will do

I'm sorry I don't wear her face

I'm sorry I don't bare her name
I'm sorry I'm not what you need
But I love you, all the same

~*~

    Blair had a band for a while called The Urban Folk
Collective made up of him, Dale, Ken Comstock, Afeni Ngozi Hill,
and either Chris Winter on drums, or Eric "Other" Jilson on
turntables/production. The members rotated a little bit, but
the show they put on was always amazing. I remember going to
one of their cd release parties at The Magic Stick, a concert
venue downtown, and you would have thought I was going to
prom. I spent all day getting ready for that show, and I
remember what I wore: black slacks with the foot high boots I
had recently stolen with a very fitted white button-down
collared shirt underneath a black cummerbund and a black neck
tie, untied, with my shirt unbuttoned enough to let my girls
show. I had dark make-up on, and a black scarf in my still very
short hair as I had just shaved off my first set of dreadlocks only
a few months prior. My favorite pretty boy gave me a lap dance
and I think a few of us had a bit too much to drink; but the night
made for a good story I don't remember so well, and would
probably be discouraged from telling if I did.

    A few weeks later, Leah and I went to City Club, a Goth
Industrial club in downtown Detroit at Cass and Bagley. We
needed our ID and cover money to get in so we brought that
with us, but we left our purses in the car, which hers had her
phone in it, and mine had my journal, the one I mentioned
earlier, with everything I'd ever written in it, my list of quotes
and funny moments, and the autograph of my favorite musician
at the time, John Mayer, on the back. Yes, we being silly, stupid
naïve little suburban girls, left our purses, under the seat mind
you, in a car with a back window that unzipped, in downtown
Detroit. You can see where this is going. When we came out of

the club a few hours later we found the back window unzipped, the purses missing and the driver side door open. We filed a police report, but of course the purses were never found. We called our phones the next day from my house and we were going to go get them ourselves, but thankfully, we thought better of it and let my dad know what happened and he took us. The people that had them by this point had clearly bought them off other people who bought them off other people and I think we paid maybe $30 a piece to get them back. I wanted so badly to be angry at whomever had stolen my journal because it wasn't worth pennies on the street, but meant everything to me. I knew I'd deserved it though. This is when I learned that Karma is very real, and she is a cold hearted bitch. I haven't even taken a penny candy since.

The following autumn I started a job at a chain café and sandwich shop called Cosi that was attached to a book store on one side with an arcade I had been to many times with Steve on the other side of the alley. I was a barista for quite a while, and let me tell you, people in Farmington are VERY particular about their coffee. I had one lady that came in very regularly and she would spell out her complicated but never changing drink to me in the most condescending tone of voice, as if I hadn't made it for her a hundred times and couldn't possibly remember what it was. One day she came in and did this in her usual tone, and I, in my typical friendly and always professional manner made her drink quickly and efficiently and wished her a lovely afternoon. Five minutes later, she came back up to the counter with it spilled all down her front and in an even ruder tone asked me "are you having a problem with cups and lids today?" as if it were my fault she had spilled her drink. After I explained that no, this was the first I'd heard of it, but I would certainly remake her drink for her, she then demanded I do so, and respelled it out for me as if I hadn't just made it for her five minutes prior, in that tone of hers, so I spit in it. Yes, I did. It was not my proudest moment, but it sure did make me feel better. This was the only time I ever spit in a customer's order, or even served anything questionable as far as I remember, but this lady was rude, and I don't like rude people, and I'm sure she didn't even notice.

The Barista Poem*2002
(Spoken word piece)

Hi.
My name is Jeni, and I...........
am a barista.

Not an alcoholic, a crackfiend, speedfreak, republican, net-head, midnight-toker, or even, depending who you ask, a nympho, clepto, or smoker.

I simply.........
.........................make the coffee.

I supply the fix to all the caffeine junkies and the left-over, wanna-be beatniks who need an image boost.

As of two months ago, I didn't even *like* coffee, and I sure as hell didn't *speak* it,

But when there is such a thing as free lunch, you eat.
And when there are upper middle class yuppies barking at you all day long
you learn the language.

You have to know it inside and out because half of them don't even know what the hell they're trying to say, and two thirds of those are going to pretend they are completely aware; and it will always be your fault when a mistake is made no matter where the error occurred, it is still, indeed, your fault. (Hence the button "server error" on the register. Have you ever seen the "customer is a dumbshit button? I rest my case.)

When they order an iced mocha, when in reality, they want a
frozen mocha
it is you who should have known full well what they desired.
To hell with learning the language, just read minds!

And yes, iced and frozen are two completely different concepts,
as are single, double and so forth,
regular and decaf,
whole, skim, soy and breve!

It's really very simple.
If you do not specify, you will get the default beverage.
Whole........regular.......hot.

If you still don't like it, might I suggest you take your ass to
Starbucks.
They will at least make you a coconut frappuccinno.

I, on the other hand
will not.

I will, however, charge you extra for being stupid
and will absolutely charge you double for stupid orders!

No, you may not have a gigante, no foam, decaf latte!
I did not wake my ass up at the crack of too damned early to
open this store at six in the morning so you could order nothing
but a cup of HOT MILK!
Maybe if you wanted a quad Americano, or if it were obvious
you just got off the graveyard shift and just have a thing for
overpriced sedatives
then maybe I could justify this order
but not for you to go next door to Barnes and Noble, turn on
your Kenny G.
and "wake up" to your decaf latte!
Why don't I just throw in a few sominex for you?!
(I could still be sleeping for crying out loud.)

And NO! You may not have a skim, decaf, sugarfree vanilla steamer!
This drink tastes like ass!!!
There is no fat, no caffeine, no sugar, and sure as shit no flavor!
There is absolutely no logical reason for you to ingest this beverage
And therefor, no reason for me to make it.
(Get the hell out of my store.)

And yes, bitch, your fat free caramel mocha cappuccino is indeed, fat free.
Here is the chocolate syrup: fat free.
Here is the caramel flavoring: fat free.
Here is the skim milk that I personally removed all of the fat from before steaming to make your lame-ass drink, and even the whipped cream is fucking FAT FREE!
Please do not sue the restaurant. You do not need to rearrange your entire week of weight watchers points to compensate for the zero grams of fat in your coffee.
(You might want to consider our signature salad instead of that triple cheese pizza, but hell, what do I know, I'm just the barista.)

Yes, I will make your doppio machiatto, because it's early.
And yes, I will make your wildberry smoothie, because you're cute.
But you sir, may absolutely NOT have a mint mocha with your broccoli and cheese furtada because that is gross. And no, little girl, you really don't want a frozen s'more because between you and me, honey, no one wants little bits of marshmallow swimming around their drink, and ground graham crackers? I can't do it. It's against my religion. I'm sorry.
(You're all gonna burn in hell, I swear it.)

And for the love of everything good and evil,
PLEASE!
DO NOT ATTACK THE BARISTA!!

Do not feed the barista
Do not complain to the barista
Do not hit on the barista
and do not, I REPEAT, do NOT, under any circumstances
proceed to tell the barista your entire life story.

Frankly, *I don't care* what you had for breakfast and
Frankly, *I don't care* what your co-workers are up to and
Frankly, *I don't care* whom you suspect your boyfriend is seeing
behind your back.

I am here to take your order   -
take your money
make your beverage
give you a smile
and send you on your way!

Nowhere in my job description was I informed that I'm
supposed to give a damn about your day.
I am the barista. The BARISTA!

Not hooker
Not therapist
Not friend, or beloved helpless pet.

I am not here to solve your problems.
I am not here to help you find your place in this world.
And I am not here to tell you the meaning of life.

I am simply here to blend the ice
steam the milk
and brew the coffee.

This is what I do.
I am simply, the barista.

Now get the hell out of my store.

~*~

This job is also where I met Chriggy and Schneider, my two best girls for a year or so. We called ourselves "the trio" as any group of three normally does, and we used to hang out constantly, and drink more than any underage person should. If you've seen the movie "Waiting," it was very much like that. Most restaurants are, as far as I can tell, and I've worked in quite a few by now. We went mini-golfing, drunk. We went bowling, drunk. We just went to the bowling alley and got drunk in the parking lot once and didn't even go in. This was not a fun night for me as I got very sick and vomited just from the smell of the burger joint across the street. There were several nights I just slept in my car in the parking lot because I had to open the next morning. How I did this I have no idea, because I certainly couldn't anymore. It was only ten years ago, but I honestly think I would die if I tried half of it now.

We made up this "language" like pig-Latin, or Ithig, or whatever the kids are doing these days where we would throw the sound "iggity" into the middle of the word. Why did we do this? Who knows?! But it was our thing. There were four different Jenny's at our Cosi, so we gave them each nick-names. I think one was "hostess Jeni," one was "Oren's Jenny" (for a bit, until they broke up, and then I slept with Oren,) I don't remember the other one, and I was lovingly nick-named "Slut Jeni," which of course was shortened to "Sliggity Jiggity," and then just "Slig Jig." It may very well have been my own idea to call me this, I'm really not sure. I was proud of my sexual freedom and didn't care who knew it. My theory was, as long as you're open and honest with people, and you USE PROTECTION, there's nothing wrong with a little playtime. I will admit though, I think I may have broken a heart or two. Not that I'm Miss Thang, or some magical perfect woman, but it did get back to me that a few of my suitors felt used, which was never my intention. I was young and ignorant and foolishly assumed that all men just wanted casual flings; and for this, I am sorry.

One of my best stories was the summer after my freshman year at Michigan State, I was flying out to Orange County, California to visit my Aunt Jan and then very young cousins, Michael and Collin. On the way back, I had a layover in Denver, Colorado where a former camp friend had recently moved to for the mountains as he was an avid snowboarder. We had kept in touch through email and social media and whatnot, and had become rather flirtatious, but hadn't seen each other in many years, since before I had even discovered my sexual side. Before my trip I called him up, asked if he'd be up for some company for a few hours, and then called the airline to see if I could change my flight. They explained that this would incur a fairly substantial fee; so I asked "so if I happen to miss my connecting flight, what happens at that point?" Obviously, the customer service representative knew what I was really asking, but she had to politely tell me that I would be booked on the next flight out, for free. So, being that my connection was only 30 minutes out, I waited until I had missed it, went up to the counter (teddy bear in hand, of course) and cried to the woman that my watch was still on California time and I missed my flight, whatever would I do?! And she booked me on the next flight out to Detroit, four hours later. Being that my friend only lived about a half hour from the airport, this was more than enough time.

Maybe Baby*2004

Maybe if my eyes were just a little bluer
Or maybe if my lies were just a little truer
Maybe if my thighs were just a little smoother
Maybe if I were less a dreamer, more a doer

Maybe if my skin was just a little darker
Or maybe if my tits were just a little larger
Maybe if my tummy was just a little more toned
If you had a warm meal on your table every night when you got
home

Then maybe baby, maybe baby
Maybe baby
Would you want me then?

Maybe if my feet were just a little smaller
Or maybe if I could just be just a little bit taller
Maybe if my legs were just a little longer
Or maybe if I could just be just a little bit stronger

Maybe if my teeth were just a little whiter
Or maybe if I were less a lover more a fighter
Maybe if I was just a little better writer
Or maybe if my ass was just a little tighter

Then maybe baby, maybe baby
Maybe baby
Would you want me then?

Then maybe baby, maybe baby
Maybe baby
Would you want me then?

Maybe if I picked up your shirts from the dry cleaners
Or maybe if I could keep your house a little neater
Maybe if my lips were just a little sweeter
If I could erase my past so I had never been a cheater

But then again.....

Maybe if you would ever let me out the kitchen
Maybe if when I'm speakin you were actually listenin
Maybe if you could bring home even half the bacon
Or maybe if every night I didn't need be fakin...

Then maybe baby, maybe baby
Maybe baby
I might want you then

Maybe baby, maybe baby
Maybe baby
I might want you then...

~*~

One summer we took a road trip out to New York for what
was supposed to be this amazing two-day, thirty five artist line-
up music festival called Field Day Fest. We didn't find out until
the week of, however, that they didn't secure the permits for
the field in time, and didn't think they were going to have
enough security. It was moved to the Meadowlands stadium in
New Jersey, cut down to only one day, the list of artists was cut
to only sixteen, but most of the bands we wanted to see were
still playing; like Beck, The Beastie Boys and Radiohead, so we
still w)ent. The day of the concert was chilly, it rained all day,
everything was wet, and Beck was knocked down a flight of
stairs and rushed to the hospital just before his set, so he didn't
perform. Then the Beastie Boys had horrible sound issues and
by the time Radiohead came on to close out the night, the
whole thing was such a bummer, but they still put on an
amazing show.

We still stayed the extra day in New York and walked
around Manhattan. That night we decided we wanted to drink
in our hotel room, but were all underage and just decided to try
buying beer from a drugstore that shall remain nameless, and
because I was the oldest, I brought the case up to the counter,
showed the cashier my ID when asked, paid the man and left.
We just assumed he didn't really care but knew he was on
camera and had to ask and may or may not have even looked at
my birthday, because honestly, who hands over their ID if they

know they're underage? Yup. This girl. We went back to our crappy hotel room at a rather large discount hotel chain that will also remain nameless because we were promised two beds and then given only one double that all three of us were trying to cram into, and proceeded to get slightly inebriated. All in all, this was a very fun trip.

It went on like this a few more years, constant open-mics and shows of friends and their bands. My dad let me transfer to Wayne State for my sophomore year, but my dumb ass got into a pretty bad car accident on my way to auditioning for a musical and totaled my tracker. Damn, I miss that car. So, instead of being able to live downtown, my dad said he would buy me a new car, (and by "new" I mean a thousand dollar piece of junk with major transmission issues, but I still appreciated the gesture) but I had to live at home. This was probably better because if I didn't have someone around to tell me to go to class, I probably wouldn't have. I think I had more credits in one semester at State than I ended up with my entire sophomore year at Wayne.

In early November, Leah and I went to a party at Blair's, where we met Ross. Ross was not unattractive, and he had a fancy red BMW and gauges in his ears, but Leah got to him first. No biggie. She and I were headed up to Starbucks, where he worked, a few weeks later for a visit, where we met Eric, one of Ross's friends who was also waiting for him to get off. I know it's very romantic to be all like "I knew right then and there that this was the man I was going to marry," but it would be a complete lie if I said that here, and I'm sure he would agree. I knew as soon as I met him that I was going to go home with him because he had the sexiest voice I'd ever heard, but I was only nineteen when we met and I was still convinced I was never going to get married in those days.

A few days later we all met up at The Music Menu in Greektown where another great local band had a Thursday night residency, The Brothers Groove. We did a bunch of

Lemon Drops and danced, and Leah made up some story about some people they ran into or something so that I would go home with Eric, but that was already my plan, so I'm still a little unclear what happened there, but long story short, Eric and I started dating, and shortly thereafter, even moved in together.

He was a House DJ by night, a really good one that had learned a lot from Chicago greats during his stay out there and he was putting together a demo, trying to book parties and we had talked about moving back out there when I was done with school. My big mouth had to ask him one day "if you were offered a house gig out in Chicago, today, would you take it?" knowing full well that would mean I wouldn't be coming along because I had to finish school and couldn't afford out of state tuition. He initially said no, but I guess he thought about it some more and a few days later he came home and said "we need to talk." I wrote many songs in the months that followed that break-up. This was also the last time I asked a question without thinking about if I really wanted the answer.

We Need to Talk*2003

You'll sit me on the bed
And hold my hands in yours
Look me in the eye
And pretend you're hurting too
And when you're feeling guilty
You'll hold me when I cry
And that's when you'll convince me
That it's not me, It's you

You'll spoon-feed me the bullshit
That I swallow every time
As I savor the taste
Of defeat in my mouth
Stumble and you'll stutter

Trying to find the perfect words
But they all mean the same damned thing
When they finally come out

We need to talk
We need to talk
We need to talk
We need……..

Don't tell me it's not working
Don't tell me it's not my fault
Don't tell me you've got dreams
Goddamnit, don't we all
I guess yours are more important
Though my heart is on the line
But I'm the idiot who put it there
So I guess the fault's all mine

We need to talk
We need to talk
We need to talk
We need...

If you loved me in the beginning
You'd still love me 'til the end
Don't try to tell me differently
Now all you want's a "friend"
Spare me your fucking pity
Go waste someone else's time
Find another heart to break
I'm tired of fixing mine

No, we don't need to talk
No, we don't need to talk
No, we don't need to talk
No, we don't need….

~*~

A Bird May Love a Fish*2003

Doctor, please help me
I need to be flying up there
But in place of my wings
Are these funny webbed things
And I can't seem to breathe the air

And Oh, my love's going to leave me
Because we can't find a common ground
She nests in the trees
And I'm stuck in the seas
I'm so sick of swimming around

So drop me a postcard
When you get to Belize
I'll save you some sand
From each of the seas
And if I had any of my own
I would fall on my knees
And beg God, to give me some wings
Oh, please God, won't you give me
Some wings

Doctor, please hurry
I think I'm running out of time
She's bored with my love
It's no longer enough
I think she's going to leave me behind

Doctor, I'm so worried
I really think I'm losing my girl
Why didn't I listen
When they said we're from two different worlds

So drop me a postcard
When you get to Belize

I'll save you some sand
From each of the seas
And if I had any of my own
I would fall on my knees
And beg God, to give me some wings
Oh, please God, won't you give me
Some wings

Doctor, No thank you
Please take these little pills back
I've realized I don't need a disguise
I'd rather just be who I am

It's not meant to be
If she can't love me for me
And we can't find a compromise
But let truth be told
Need I be so bold
I shouldn't have to change my life

When you perch on the Eiffel
And you look to the blue
When you see my waters
You'll know I'm missing you
I'm sorry I'm not the thing
That you needed me to be
But I'm not sorry for being me

So drop me a postcard
When you get to Belize
I'll save you some sand
From each of the seas
And if I had any of my own
I would fall on my knees
And thank God for not giving me wings
Oh, thank God, for not giving me wings...

~*~

Dreamer's Lullaby*2003

When the weight of the world
Is crushing you down
There's no use in removing
Your head from those clouds
When you'll always regret
Taking the easy way out
And giving up on the jeweled life
You'd otherwise have found

The road to the emerald city
Isn't always paved in gold
The path may be dark and winding
And heavy will be your load
But look how far you've come by now
To give up and turn around
When you've already lost so much
There's so much you haven't yet found

There's door number one
Or door number two
A choice to be made
And neither's wrong or right
When one makes you happy
And the other's just easy
If you turn from your dreams
Can you sleep through the night?

How can you sleep without your dreams
How can you sleep without your dreams
How can you sleep...
How can you sleep...

~*~

The following May I threw a birthday show for what was really my twentieth birthday, but I told the bar where I was throwing it that it was my twenty-first birthday, and no one ever asked me for ID. I was in there all the time for their Tuesday open-mics, also hosted by Blair, so they knew me anyway. I played a short set, as did Dale, Dan Minard, and Ian Lee Lamb. Everyone that I wanted to be there that night was there, and it was another highlight of my life. All of my favorite people and music for my birthday, it was lovely.

The next day I got a call from a boy in one of my classes that I had seen around at open-mics and was friends with Blair, and "in the scene" if you will. I was at work, but he left me a message I saved for a long time saying what a wonderful party I'd thrown and he would want his exactly the same way. I had a mini crush on this boy, but he had a girlfriend, so I just assumed he was off limits. Another long story short: they were having problems, they broke up, we got together, in that order. I was not a home-wrecker. Yet.

His name was Matt and we dated almost three years. I don't know if I ever told him this, but I attribute my graduating Wayne State to him. He took a few classes with me that he had no business taking as a Public Relations major, including Design 2: Color Theory, the most difficult class I took. He would stay up all night with me while we worked on these poster sized journals and painting exercises trying to mix the exact right shade, or hue, or tint, or whatever the hell it was supposed to be that was never right! That professor definitely made me cry a few times. I needed this class for my art major but I feel like I may have dropped it and changed majors all together if it weren't for Matt.

Coward*2003

It feels just like I've been sleeping

But I can't seem to wake
And I know my body must be screaming
But no one comes to my aid
And I know the morning is coming
To wake me up with a kiss
But Oh how I wish she'd hurry
I can't go on like this

Fear of those nights
Fear of those mornings
Fear of the aching that never subsides
Fear of those days
Feeling like nothing
The fear of losing my will
To survive

And you just might be perfect
The dream that I let slip away
But I'll never know all I lost to the wind
Because I was too afraid
If only I could close my eyes
To all that I have seen
Then maybe I could finally learn
To just let a dream be a dream
They're all nightmares to me
All nightmares to me

Afraid of those nights
Afraid of those mornings
Afraid of the aching that never subsides
Afraid of those days
Feeling like nothing
Afraid of losing my will too survive

Afraid of the dark
Afraid of the lonely
Afraid of love lost as it trickles to the floor
Afraid of the razor making love to my skin

Because I can't love
Anymore
Can't love anymore…

Love me, teach me to be unafraid
Love me, and frighten my fears away
Love me, and say you'll understand
Love me for the coward that I am

Fear of those nights
Fear of those mornings
Fear of the aching that never subsides
Fear of those days
Feeling like nothing
The fear of losing my will
To survive

~*~

     I heard a statistic when I was first starting school that the average college student has seven different majors before they graduate, which I thought was absurd; until I had eight. I was undecided for the first semester at Michigan State, then I decided to be theatre, then it was fashion design, then interior design, then graphic design, video arts, studio art with a concentration in drawing and painting and ultimately: printmaking. Funny thing is, I honestly didn't even know what printmaking was until I was invited (as a graphic design major) to a meeting to review the new Wayne State website before it launched. I just happened to sit down next to Stanley, the head of the Printmaking department, who looked as much like Santa Claus as one could without a red suit and reindeer. He commented that I had very nice handwriting and that I should take his etching class. So the next semester, I did, and I liked it. And I liked Stanley. I thought I could definitely take more classes from this man, and I didn't particularly care for drawing and painting all that much the way it was being taught. It's unfortunate I wasn't able to get into a screen printing class until my senior year because this turned out to be my true love. As long as it was flat, or could be flexed to be flat, you could print on it, and I just started printing on everything! The stool at my desk in the communal studio, t-shirts, bandannas, CD cases and even toilet seats. These became my signature piece as I found a local hardware store where I could buy them for five dollars, disassemble them, paint them, print them, and then giftwrap them back up and sell them for thirty dollars at art fairs. Detroit was great for this sort of thing because there were always art fairs, always artists looking to split booth rental, and always people interested in buying cheap, kitschy, art.

I actually hated being a studio art major, but it was already my senior year by the time I made this decision, and I wasn't about to stay in school forever, at that time anyway. All the professors wanted me to talk about my work like "what I'm trying to say with this piece is..." or "this piece says to the world that..." and blah blah blah, bullshit. I didn't have a statement to make. I just wanted to make things pretty. I loved bright swirling colors, and glitter, and generally felt driven to make the world a prettier place, but I had no "statement". I did a whole series of prints for my senior project about not being an artist. Bright, beautiful prints (in my opinion anyway) with bold wording saying "this is not art" and "I am not an artist" or one of my personal favorites, the sarcastic "I have a statement!" Stanley said I would make more money than anyone else, and perhaps I would have if I'd stuck with it, but unfortunately, real life took over. I know everyone says do what you love and you'll never work a day in your life or some crap, but rent doesn't pay itself and once I graduated, Daddy stopped paying it, so I went back to Cosi.

I applied for a tattoo apprenticeship at one point, and was offered the position after an extensive interview and portfolio review; but they wanted me to work in their shop for about thirty hours a week, unpaid, in exchange for my training and equipment costs, and I was already working forty hours or thereabouts at Cosi, so I turned it down. This is one of the decisions I feel like probably had a great impact on which direction my life took. I think next time around I'll take it.

The other thing I don't know how I would have gotten through without Matt, was my dad moving to Jacksonville, Florida. As I mentioned earlier, he had quit Compuware some years ago and was working from home and living off of stock market winnings. As soon as my brother graduated high school though, in 2003, he sold our house and we moved to Ferndale, a nice enough, highly rentable city right on the northern border of Detroit. It was also only a few blocks from Woodward Avenue which ran straight through the center of Ferndale, and all the way down through the center of Detroit, where Wayne State was, so that my brother could take the bus home on the weekends if he so chose, but I think he usually just hitched a ride with me.

In any case, the money was running out, and he had casually mentioned needing to get a job soon, but one day I came home from class and he had an interview in Jacksonville in two days. He flew down, interviewed, drove around in his rental car for a day or two looking for a rental house, flew back, packed up the necessary items, and Matt and I drove his car while he drove the moving truck. He flew us back within a day or two. All of this happened inside the span of two weeks and let me tell you, I was a mess. I had a pretty good idea how close I was to my dad and how much I would miss him once he was no longer around all the time, but you would have thought he died the way I moped around after the fact. I remember Matt's mom asked me about a week later how I was doing and I just lost it; just broke down sobbing! It was bad. But, like everything else, I got over it. Matt's parents liked to take road trips with us, so we just started adding Jacksonville, Florida to the route, even though it's about eleven hundred miles and a good sixteen hour drive from Detroit, but they would trade driving and we would sleep, and everyone had a great time.

Matt and I stayed in the Ferndale house as my dad had already paid for the whole year in advance, and we rented out a room to Dale, who helped us turn the bungalow room upstairs into a pretty awesome recording studio. I put out a little four track EP, Dale recorded a whole bunch of things with a bunch of different friends, and the local band Tone and Niche recorded the whole album "On the Streets of" at my house. We also designed all of their jacket sleeves, their press boxes, printed their discs, designed the programs and fliers for the release show, and I was one of the opening acts, performing with our friend, Rod, and his band. This was the only time I performed my own material with a full band and It. Was. Awesome.

It was also around this time that Dale and Dan Minard sat me down and opened my eyes to the fact that my appearance didn't fit my music at all. I had never really thought about it, but I wore crazy bright colors, tie-dye, hippie floral prints, bell bottoms, and had brightly colored hair that frequently changed colors. I was bright and happy. My music, on the other hand, was not. My artwork was always brightly colored and glittery, but my songs were depressing and we all used to joke that I should be sponsored by Kleenex and my albums should come with a free pack of tissues. My slogan was "taking over the world, one tear at a time." My songs are generally slow and melodic and about heartbreaks and hardships. The perfect example is the story behind "Eva's Song." When I decided to write it, I was determined to write a happy song because I didn't have any. I thought of the happiest time in my life, which was the summer between high school and college when I was in Rimers of Eldritch and I decided to write a song from Eva's perspective; but (as I mentioned earlier) her best friend tries to rape her in the end. It was by far the most depressing song I'd ever written at that point.

They really set me straight that yes, although it's kind of

selling out to change your image to sell your music, fact of the matter is, if you want to make money selling records, your image should probably match your music. So, the next day I died my hair black and started wearing more dark colors and darker makeup and fell more into the Goth stereotype for a quite a while.

Eva's Song*2004

Here I sit, every hour, every day
Mama braids my hair, but I never go play
Just stay in the house, where I know that it's safe
And no one can take me away

Betrayed, by the one I trusted most
Never saw it coming, one day he just let go
In a flash of trees, I fell to the ground
And no one can save me now

Policeman asks me questions, but I just sit and stare
I swear I can't remember, but I swear he just don't care
I don't remember screaming, and I hope I never will
All I know is that time stood still

I haven't shed a tear, I haven't said a word
I haven't shut my eyes since the day I tasted dirt
With these scars of leaves and needles now eternal on my face
Here is where I'll stay

~*~

CHAPTER 5

After the lease on that house was up, Matt and I moved down to an apartment near campus that Tom and his girlfriend moved into as well. I loved living downtown. I loved that apartment. It had a lot of charm, including the separate faucets for hot and cold water in the bathroom, which only looks cool but is really a pain, a claw foot tub, and the longest hallway with floorboards that could wake the dead. I did a lot of my best work during this year, my senior year, living in this apartment. I got into a few art shows, I built a really strong portfolio, and even got paid for a couple of design jobs and mural painting gigs. My favorite was the Street Painting, or "Madonnari" exhibition during the Festival of the Arts that I did for three years. I had to submit an idea, be selected by a panel of judges, and then they would supply the artists with a box of pastels and a taped off ten foot square in the roped off street, and we had three days to recreate our murals in the street with the pastels. I loved it. Who wouldn't love being paid a few hundred dollars to essentially play with sidewalk chalk?

But alas, eventually I did graduate, and the lease was up on that apartment, so Matt and I moved in with our friend, Rod. Problem was, Rod was technically Matt's superior at work now, and one of the others in the office that no one liked, squealed.

Fortunately, the higher bossman was kind about it and pulled Matt aside and gave him a month to move out, and did not fire him, but it was still a royal pain moving twice in only a couple months. I mean, don't get me wrong, I think I'm the only person in the world that actually loves moving, and have done A LOT of it, but it's still kind of a process, and a bit expensive, and our rent nearly doubled from what we were paying Rod to live with him.

This was also the first time I had lived alone with just Matt. At Wayne State, my brother and his girlfriend were living with us, and before that it was back and forth from my dad's house, to his parents' house. Matt and I were already having issues, and I was terrified of commitment, and living together just the two of us just felt so overwhelmingly domestic, and I'm sorry to say, old. I was still immature. I wanted to go back to school and stay young and keep partying, and like my teenage years, I did not handle the "welcome to the real world" very well either.

Forbidden Fruit*2005

I can see it, through the window
Shiny brand new toy
So much bigger and better
Than playthings previously enjoyed

Mommy is saying not this time
Come on now, come along
But I am only human
Have desires even when I know they're wrong

So I give into temptation
Watch the world come crashing down
Forbidden fruits taste so much sweeter
Than those that we're allowed

Can you see it, how it sparkles
It's really caught my eye
Yes I remember, I promised no more toys
Please just this one last time

Mommy, please can I get it
I know the price is kinda high
I'll return it in the morning
Let me play for just one night

So let's give into temptation
Watch the world come crashing down
Forbidden fruits taste so much sweeter
Than those that we're allowed

~*~

      After Eric and I had broken up, we stayed in contact, and actually became very good friends. He started dating another girl while I was dating Matt, and we were completely platonic and quite literally just friends for a few years. I even remember driving with Blair somewhere and him asking me if Matt and I ever broke up if I thought I would get back together with Eric, and I really believed what I said when I explained that I really didn't think so. But Blair knew everything, and he just got this look on his face that I didn't question. I'm sure you can see where this is going. Rod helped Matt get a better job with the Wayne State Library System, working evenings. Eric and I were already hanging out here and there, but once Matt was gone until ten at night most the time, I started going to Eric's more regularly, and well, you can put the pieces together for yourself. The unfortunate element is that Matt always knew where I was, I never even lied to him. Poor Matt was just so trusting, and I just threw it in his face. Pretty slut move that I am not exactly proud of.

Raspberry Swirl*2005

Why'd you have to whisper the words
We were never supposed to say
Why couldn't you just leave sleeping dogs
Alone to dream away
You've stirred them from their slumber
Now all they want to do is play
Good job, way to go
You've ruined everything

'Cause you're so tempting
And confident
And he's so safe
And vanilla
And you are milk chocolate
And raspberry swirl
And I'm just a selfish little girl

How could you let me come over
And just give myself to you
When you know that I've promised another
To love him and always be true
But now that you've caught me, I can' turn away
From the entrapment in your eyes
Anyway, what kind of woman would I be
If my cravings went denied

'Cause you're so tempting
And confident
And he's so safe
And vanilla
And you are milk chocolate
And raspberry swirl
And I'm just a selfish little girl

And this time is the last time
I can't do this anymore
I know I said this last time
And all the times before
He deserves much better
Than a liar and a cheat
But Goddamn I can't help the way
That you enrapture me

'Cause you're so tempting
And confident
And he's so safe
And vanilla
And you are milk chocolate
And raspberry swirl
And I'm just a selfish little girl

~*~

The bigger twist to this story is that Eric was in kinda a tight spot with money at that time, and his rent was about to go up. Matt, obviously having no idea I had already slept with him again, suggested he move in with us. It would help Eric save money, it would help me feel less domestic and settled, it was the best of both worlds. You're cringing now, aren't you? So, New Year's Day, 2006, the day after my mother left from one of her visits, Eric moved into our spare room. Needless to say, Eric and I were like bunnies. The cheating element was so exciting. I think Matt must have just been in denial. This only lasted a couple months before I finally snapped and couldn't do it anymore and broke up with Matt, hoping he would never find out about Eric. Oh how naïve I still was.

Blair had become a very good friend of mine, and was great to talk to because he was such a good listener, and he had this policy of never assuming he knew everything about someone else's relationship no matter how much they'd told him because there were always little nuances and details that get left out, and wouldn't offer advice unless asked for it. So, he was the only one that knew I was sleeping with Eric. He was also a good friend of Matt's, but he swore to me everything I told him was between me and him and it was no business of his to come between us. Shortly after Matt and I had broken up, but before I had moved out of our house I wrote a very long email to Blair about what was going on, what I was feeling, what my plans were, etc. etc. and to this day, Matt swears Blair "accidentally" forwarded the email to him, which I refuse to believe. Blair would never do such a thing and then lie to my face when I asked him. He might do it and then tell me he did, but I am convinced Matt hacked Blair's email, or my email. He had the computer knowledge, or access to a keystroke tracking program through work, and I had heard Matt lie to people all the time about other things he had dropped the ball on, so it was always someone else's fault. But he came away from our computer and just said to me "what happened with Eric" and so I told him.

Wishing Well*2006

I've taken six or seven bottles worth of Diphenhydramine
Eaten eleven or twelve gallons worth of cookie dough ice cream
About a thousand pounds of chocolate every couple days
Still nothing makes the pain go away

I try to wash my sorrows down with Johnny, Jack and Jim
By day after tomorrow I'll have healed these etchings in my skin
I've driven back and forth nine times from New York to L.A.
Still nothing makes the pain go away

I've thrown every cent I ever earned down every wishing well
Tried to bargain with the devil, but had no soul left to sell
And It's been years since I've known faith, but I dropped to my

knees and prayed
Still nothing makes the pain go away

Every morning I awaken and fight back the need to cry
I stand in the mirror, try to hold my head up high
I swear that I'll get through this live to fight another day
Still nothing makes the pain go away

No nothing makes the pain
Go away

~*~

Fortunately, I was only around for one more week of awkwardness. I didn't know if I wanted to be with Eric full time at that moment; I wasn't even positive I didn't want to be with Matt; but I think that was just the discomfort of a breakup looming. I was really thinking about just being single for a while, and my dad was totally cool with me coming to stay with him in Florida for however long I needed to figure it out. Problem with this plan is that my dad was now working full time, and as cool as he was, I could only go to the bar with him so many times before I really needed to start branching out and meeting some people my own age, which I did not do the whole three months I was there. I pretty much stayed in the house, designed a website, and sold some printed shirts on Ebay.

Novelty*2006

I wear bright colors, I am small
My eyes they sparkle like the sand
I'm cute and clever, I've got it all
I clutch your fingers in my little hand

Summerwalk barefoot down the street
When autumn's falling I collect the leaves
Winterdance angels in the snow
When springtime's blooming I'm a child like nobody knows

You think I'm cute
You think I'm charismatic
I'm a ray of sunshine
I am bloody fantastic
But the things that you see
Have got nothing to do with me
And I can't be your novelty

I cry whenever I'm alone
Can't stand to see my own reflection
It's been so long since I've been home
Can't heal these scars of past rejections

You kiss my lips and hold my hand
But you have no idea who I really am
When you start to learn what makes me tick
Just like the others, you'll grow sick
and tired of me

You think I'm cute
You think I'm charismatic
I'm a ray of sunshine
I am bloody fantastic
But the things that you see
Have got nothing to do with me
And I can't be your novelty

My heart is black
My Body's made of plastic
I'm a bloody wind-up
My soul is automatic

Can't taste my lips

Can't feel my heart
It won't stop beating cuz I
Never let it start
I do not feel
I do not breathe
Go ahead and cut me, you can watch
While I don't bleed

I am not cute
I am not charismatic
I'm a fucking raincloud
I am monochromatic

All that I let you see
Has got nothing to do with me
And I'm sorry
But I can't be your novelty

~*~

Eric called me every day. We would talk for hours. He was clearly in love with me and wanted me to come back. He visited a few times. The first time we drove down to Daytona Beach for a few days, and the second time we met in Atlanta. It was on this trip to Atlanta that I got a phone call about a job in Jacksonville that I had applied for, a graphic design job. It was a full time, salaried job that I very stupidly told the man I didn't even know if I was qualified for. His exact words were "that's okay, we can train you in anything you don't know. You just have such a sparkling personality, I'd love to add you to our team." I was already thinking about moving back home though, and I didn't want to take the job away from someone else who needed one. This is another decision I wonder about. How different would my life be now if I'd taken that job and just stayed in Jacksonville then?

Once I realized I wasn't even going to take a full time job, I figured I should probably just get my ass in gear and get back to Michigan. I stayed for the rest of the month as I had a two week contract job lined up selling Karaoke machines at Costco. Best. Job. Ever. This company, LeadSinger Karaoke, would hire people who could sing to stand in the entrance to Costco Warehouse stores and demonstrate these karaoke microphones that plugged right into the television with RCA cables (probably USB cables now, if they're still around, this was before flatscreens). They really made their money on the chips you could buy that would plug right into the microphone which were priced up to a hundred dollars! You could hire in to the company full time, but then they had to pay your travel expenses, so they had very few of those positions available and tried to just find people locally. In 2006, fifteen dollars an hour plus seven percent commission was pretty good money for a lost puppy. It was enough to ship my stuff back to Michigan and pay for the gas to get there, that's for sure.

I remember it rained on the day I left. I said goodbye to Oreo, the dog that had been mine since seventh grade that went with my dad when he moved; and then stopped by my dad's work to say my final goodbyes to him. I cried. I said "thanks for all the fish," which was a reference to The Hitchhiker's Guide to the Galaxy, one of his favorites, and I wrote a song about it on the way back. Yes, while I was driving, pen and paper, shame on me.

Daddy's Song*2006

I cried harder than the skies
As I drove off towards the horizon
Not even knowin, where I was goin
My eyes always were the prize on

Tired of taking two steps back

For every one that I took forward
Sun rising in the distance
Guess that's what I'm headed toward

And I know that you'll be there when I return
'Cuz I'm always gonna be your little girl

Don't yet know just what it is
That I'm running from or to
But I know wherever I may go
I'm followed by the love of you

And it might be my job right now to go explore the world
But I'm always gonna be your little girl

And daddy, I love you
So much more than words can say
You gave me a home
Taught me all I know
And gave me wings to fly away

Still gonna need my daddy
Even when I'm fully grown
Still gonna call you daddy
Even when I have children of my own

Sometimes I get naïve and think I've figured out the world
But I'm always gonna be your little girl

I know I'm always gonna be
You're little girl

~*~

I didn't have any extra money and couldn't afford to
live on my own (and would have been completely opposed to

doing so at this time) so, logically, I ended up moving in with Eric, who was now staying with our friends, Chris and Jess. I went back to work for my old boss from Cosi, but he was at Einstein Bagels now, so I went there. I continued to try to make art, and painted the windows at Einstein's a few times, but I was barely able to pay my portion of rent and utilities on what I was making, so I went back to work at Cosi in the evenings. There were plenty of days where I would wake up around 5:00am to be to Einstein's by 6:00am, would work until 2:30pm, drive to Cosi, take a nap in my car, and then go in and work from 4:00pm until 10:00pm. This eventually caught up to me and I woke up one morning, and couldn't even stand up for more than a minute without feeling like I was going to black out. I still went in to work, at 6:00am, but I requested if they didn't really need me, I'd like to go home. Apparently, they ended up getting slammed that day and then wrote nasty things about me in the manager's log, but I told them I would stay if they needed me. I knew it wasn't their fault I was suffering from exhaustion, and I have the craziest sense of work ethic. I have never called off a shift.

This is also about the time I applied to be on the TV show "Survivor," the first time. I filled out a twenty page questionnaire about who I was, what I did for a living, what my hobbies and passions were, and who I wanted to come visit me if I made it on the show. I put down Blair, my dad, and Eric. Blair was a huge "Survivor" fan as well; so much so that I remember he called me one morning, while I was in Design I class the day after the season finale and he left me a message that said "Pixie, if you see me or call me, DO NOT TELL ME WHO WON SURVIVOR! I haven't watched it yet, but I will in the next day or two." We were both diehards for the show. I sent in a silly video with the questionnaire, but I overnighted it the day before it was due, so I like to tell myself they never got it, because I never got a call.

We stayed with Chris and Jess a few more months, but

Eric ultimately decided we needed our own place and we moved into a house we couldn't really afford, a few miles over, in Berkley. Fortunately, maybe a month later, I got a promotion, at Cosi, and went there full time. I still helped out at Einstein's on Saturdays, but only for a few months. My new position at Cosi was the Catering Coordinator, and I loved it. Best restaurant position I've ever held. I generally worked about 8am til 2pm, set up all the catering, including the dessert platters, which I loved arranging, delivered it all, helped through the lunch rush when I got back, and then left. Some days there was quite a bit of catering and it was very stressful, but most days there was only a reasonable amount, and there was an hourly raise involved, and I started taking home an extra couple hundred dollars a week in tips. It was great.

The following March, Eric called me one day while I was out on a delivery and said "I need $300, but I can't tell you what it's for." Obviously, as the money handler of this relationship, I could not let this slide and eventually found out he wanted to adopt a puppy from the humane society. Now, I LOVE animals. I was even vegetarian for five years and vegan for one of them back in high school and college, and I love puppies, LOVE THEM, but I did not think it was a good time for us to be getting a dog. Eric always knew what to say to get me to see things his way and next thing I knew, we were at the humane society that night. The original pup we went to see was supposedly half German Shepherd and half Rottweiler, but I think they just tell people every dog has some German Shepherd in it because they told us the other puppies we looked at were half German Shepherd and half Chow Chow. The two we played with together were brothers of the same litter. One was very chill and almost all black. The other had way more spunk, and better coloring, and we ultimately went with him. He was a little sick though and we had to come back in a few days to finalize the adoption and take him home. It ended up being St. Patrick's Day when we brought him home. We wanted to name him something Irish accordingly. My vote was for "Whiskey" as that's what he reminded me of, when you hold a glass of whisky up to the light, the striations matched his highlights exactly. Eric wanted to name him Apollo, which isn't even Irish. It was a full week before he had a name. Eventually, we went to the Royal Oak brewery, with our friend Thommy, made a list of about twenty names, a few of which were as eccentric as Doctor Gonzo, and polled the whole bar, and ultimately, "Apollo" was chosen. I lost. But that's okay, because he is pretty much the coolest dog on the planet; I don't care what any of you say. Except for those navy seal dogs, they're super bad ass.

We lived on a corner lot in our new rental house, and the yard was fenced with chain link, so anyone walking down the sidewalk could see our whole yard as they were walking by, and it sure seemed like everyone in Berkley had a dog, and boy did they love Apollo. He was the sweetest puppy, loved people, and never barked at anything! He was so playful, and smart! He knew he wasn't supposed to chew on sticks, so he had this habit of lying in the corner of the yard, looking like he was chewing on his bone, only to find out he was really chewing on a stick hiding behind his bone. Or the time we came home from work to find a puddle of pee just outside his crate because he figured out he could lift his leg and aim it away. Never before have I been simultaneously so mad and so proud! It took probably a few months before I really fell in love with that puppy and didn't want to kill him half the time, (like when he destroyed my favorite shirt, or my phone charger, or my crocks) but now I would literally give a limb for him. He's like our child.

That spring, my brother graduated from Wayne State and we threw him a graduation BBQ in our back yard and my dad came up and stayed with us, and my mother came up from Savannah and stayed with friends because she couldn't stay in a "house of sin." Let me also interject here that she had loved Matt. He had gone out of his way to blow smoke up her ass and be the son she never had (because Tom sure wasn't going to call her and talk to her for an hour) so she loved him like her own son and I think she was more devastated than I was when we split. In her mind, it was Eric's fault, and she couldn't stand him for it. I'm sure it also didn't help that the family didn't know I was now smoking and drinking until they came to our house for the BBQ and she blamed Eric for that as well, which was also not his fault. I was already doing these things before him, I just failed to mention it on the phone because really, how do you tell your mother you started smoking and drinking, especially when she's so religious, and everything you do is a sin already. She didn't speak to him or even say "thank you" for the hospitality, or cooking, or throwing the party for her son. Eric didn't take too kindly to this and doesn't speak to her to this day.

I was making better money than I ever had, and Eric was doing pretty well, but he'd been at his current job going on five years and hadn't had a raise. He was a mechanic at a local, privately owned dealership, where he had started as basically the oil change boy who swept the floors and took out the trash but was now a certified mechanic working on vehicles. He was told he'd get a raise once he got certified, but this would have taken money away from one of the other techs, so it didn't end up happening. He got yelled at for being late, but then when he tried to go in early, he got yelled at for being TOO early. He came home one day after a particularly stressful shift and announced that he was ready for a change and thought that we should move to Jacksonville. After much discussion, we ultimately decided this is what we would do in several months when our lease was up.

We had a lot of stuff at this point in our lives and we sold it all. Furniture, studio equipment, his turntables and mixer, most of his records, a couple guitars of mine, my very expensive microphones, everything, including my car because it was black and had no air conditioning. I loved that car too. I called her "Jujubee." Apparently, people are always moving south and never moving north, so it is quite a bit more money to rent a moving truck to go south one way than it is to go north. So we just sold everything and moved down in what we could fit in his dad's minivan. I went down about a week before to scout apartments and try to find a job before we got there so we'd have somewhere to live and at least one of us would be working. My dad had since moved to Gainesville, Florida, but that was only about an hour and a half drive to Jacksonville, so he let me stay with him and borrow his car for the duration of my trip. I did manage to procure us an apartment, and me a job, with Quiznos Subs, as an assistant manager. I thought the ad said sixteen dollars per hour, but it was actually sixteen thousand per year salary. The district manager I interviewed with, Wayne, thankfully brought this up in the interview and I initially turned the job down as that was about half of what I was currently making at Cosi and I felt I could do better. He spent the next half hour drawing me a map of the city and telling me where all the best restaurants and shopping were and where to go and where to stay away from. It was super helpful and really nice. The next day he called back and told me he could start me at 24,000 and once I got promoted to full General Manager it could go up to more like 28,000, so I accepted.

CHAPTER 6

We got lucky with our apartment; it was originally going to be on the ground floor facing the parking lot, but some mix-up moved us to the second floor over-looking the lagoon area in the back for the same amount. Even though they supposedly sprayed for bugs and spiders every week, there were spiders bigger than I'd ever seen in the breezeway outside our door and I just remember hurrying in and out the door all the time.

Eric had a friend, Mike, who had moved to the South Florida area a couple years prior who came up to visit us a few weeks after we arrived. We made the very unfortunate mistake of leaving Apollo out of his crate while we went out for a few hours. I sure wish we'd taken pictures of the destruction when we returned because it was monumental! We thought we had put everything locked in the bedroom, but Eric had a backpack in the corner that got shredded, with a box of Mrs. Grass chicken noodle soup, which was all over the dining room. He also shredded two umbrellas and pulled every single vertical blind out of their clips and proceeded to shred them. I felt bad because there was blood on the blinds and I knew it was our fault for leaving him out before he was ready. He never touched a thing that wasn't his when we were home, but if we left him home alone, he was not happy about it, and he would let you know it. He would bark loud enough for China to hear him every time he went in his crate. By about five months after we moved there, a neighbor apparently complained to the office and we were essentially evicted. We had only signed a seven month lease and were planning to move anyway so they just let us move at six months instead so it wasn't a big deal, but it was still embarrassing.

We looked at several places, including a duplex I really liked with a fenced yard, but ended up in a townhouse we couldn't really afford, a running theme in our relationship. I will say, it was very nice. It was two stories with the living room open to the loft-style stairway, two big bedrooms, a kitchen larger than we ever would have needed, a dining room we almost never used, and the tiniest possible patio, which was fenced in but Apollo wouldn't even pee in because it was all rocks beyond the pavement so we still had to walk him a handful of times a day. We had so many problems with this place.

In the summer, in Florida, it rains every afternoon, usually for only twenty minutes, and then goes back to being beautiful and sunny; but our townhouse was on the end of the unit, at the lower end of a downslope, so all the water ended up on our roof, and there was apparently a crack in some seam somewhere because it poured in through our kitchen light fixture every time it rained. We let management know about this and they sent maintenance guys out a couple times, but it never fixed the issue. It continued to rain in our kitchen, and mold grew in the closets, the pantry and the air vents. Clearly, we broke the lease on this property and moved out.

For the year we were in Florida, I hated it for the first few months, I'm not going to lie about that. I missed my friends and my open-mic scene and hadn't discovered the arts and music of Jacksonville yet, and I was working a mandatory six-day work week with Quiznos. After about two months, the manager of the Riverside store got caught stealing from the company, was promptly fired, and I got his store and my first raise. I LOVED Riverside. It was just like Ferndale with little shops and cafes, a walking path through the park and along the river, with Spanish moss hanging all over everything; my kind of area. What I did not love was working so much. A week after I took over the Riverside branch, I learned my assistant manager was on the registered sex offenders list, and not for something excusable, like taking a piss in public; something unforgivable, and he had failed to mention that on his original application, so I fired him. It wouldn't have been so bad if the man I had trained and ready to take over his position hadn't stopped showing up to work two days later. I had two key holders, who knew the basics of closing, but no one that knew how to do any paperwork, inventory, ordering, scheduling, or anything else managerial but me. There was a span of five weeks that I worked every day. Most Saturdays I would go in, open up and leave within an hour or two, but all the other days were full shifts, including my weekly open to close on Tuesdays. The only good that came from this is my District Manager saw how dedicated I was and gave me a second raise after a month at that store.

Eric got a job with a flagship golf course, the headquarters of the PGA Tour, TPC Sawgrass in Ponte Vedra, Florida which was right outside Jacksonville. I never thought he'd make it because he was required to be there by 5:30am most mornings, but he surprised me. He loved it. He was always on time. Like me, he would rather go to work very early and get out early. Problem with this job though is that he worked with a lot of younger guys, and they would very frequently go to the bar when they got out of work. I'm probably exaggerating this a bit, but it sure felt like at least three days a week they would end up at Lynch's, a pretty neat little Irish pub by the beach. We definitely had some good times at Lynch's, including our collective birthday party because they're only five days apart.

The other bar that I think we spent equally, if not more time at, was Sneakers. It was a big chain sports bar where all the servers wore cheerleader outfits or jerseys. We were both smokers at this point, and they had a very nice patio bar with TV's all over that you could smoke at, while never missing a football game, which Eric is VERY into. This is where we met the majority of our Florida friends, the patio bar of the Southside location of Sneakers. I don't think any of them were even from Florida. They were all transplanted there, as more than half of Jacksonville residents were, many from Wisconsin, a couple from Pittsburgh. Eric had his Sawgrass crew, I had my Riverside crew, and we both had our Sneakers crew.

All of these people became very crucial when Eric informed me we should move back to Michigan about ten months into our stay. Initially, I agreed, but the more I thought about it, I was happy where we were. Yes, I still missed Blair and Leah and my Detroit crew, but I had made new friends and I liked the Florida weather way better. Eric and I had been having problems, we were not communicating worth a damn, and I ultimately told him I was staying in Florida. We didn't really speak for a few days other than to figure out who was going to stay in the townhouse with the dog, and who was going to crash with a friend; which was me, on Jamie's couch. This one hurt the worst so far though and we got together a few days later to try to work it out, appropriately, at Sneakers. I won't go into the details, but let's just say we each brought stipulations to the table, most were agreed to, decided to get back together and move back to Michigan. I lost that one too.

Funny side note story: When I called my mother to tell her that we were moving back to Michigan, the conversation went as follows: "I have some bad news and you're not going to like it very much" to which her reaction was "oh my God, you're getting married!" Clearly, I informed her this was not the case, and that we were only moving back to Michigan, which to her, was just as bad. I just couldn't believe that her first conclusion to jump to when I said "I have BAD news" would be that I was getting married. This is how much she still disapproved of Eric at the time.

CHAPTER 7

When we were looking for a house to move into in the Detroit area, the weirdest thing happened: our old house in Berkley was available, even though we'd only been gone about ten months. We loved this house and loved the idea of moving back in, so we called the landlords right away, who obviously, were thrilled to have us back. Remember how I said moving trucks are significantly cheaper to go north? We rented one for the way back and kept all of our crap we had purchased upon moving down. Eric drove the truck with his car on a trailer, and I drove my car and Apollo rode with me. Let me tell you, whoever thinks that dogs don't remember things more than a few minutes is out of their mind because as soon as I got off the freeway, which was still a few miles from the house, Apollo flipped out. He knew exactly where we were, and where we were going and he was so excited. When we got there he ran around and around in crazy circles for what seemed like hours.

It was very strange for me though, moving back into the same house. The lady who rented it after we left never fully moved in. The landlords told us she had her bed propped up against the wall in the dining room. There was still a cabinet full of our groceries in the kitchen, boxes of my art supplies I had left in the garage, and our Christmas tree still in the basement.

It was very surreal. It made me feel like Florida had all been a dream and didn't really happen, and all the friends I had made, I didn't really make. I remember calling Jamie that night and crying to her about the whole thing.

I had already lined up that I would be going back to Cosi, again. Yes, for the fourth time now. I was to be a salaried assistant manager now so I had to go through management training at the Birmingham store under Karen, the current Training General Manager in the Detroit market. I don't know what kind of mafia connections this bitch had, or what kind of dirt she had on whom, but there was no reason whatsoever she should have still had a job the way she treated people. She hadn't passed anyone through her training program in over a year, would scream at her associates, yell at her customers, wore blue jeans to work and flip flops around before open, which is against health code, and did all sorts of things other than work while she was on shift. She even pulled me off a shift once to go deliver a subpoena to her boyfriend's brother because she needed someone he wouldn't recognize. The questionable things Karen did are endless and I have no idea to this day why she hasn't been fired, because I fully well know that higher-ups are aware. I am convinced the only reason she passed me through is because I had already been with the company for several years in the recent future, had worked with several of the managers still there, and had a reputation for basically being the best associate since sliced bread, so I'm sure Mike, my District Manager, made it clear to Karen that I was to pass. Andrea was not so lucky however.

Andrea was another of Karen's trainees. She started only a week or two after I did, but brand new to the company. She had a hospitality degree from Michigan State and had managed a Jay Alexander's for several years before coming to Cosi. I'm sure she knew more about managing a restaurant than I did. I remember when she was interviewing, Karen said some horrible things about her and I felt drawn to do anything I could to protect her from the evil that was Karen. We became very good friends and I did what I could, but ultimately, once Karen decides someone "can't" do the job, they are let go. Karen didn't train anymore after that though. They all got put with Amy and me at the Southfield location.

I loved Amy, my new boss once I was moved over to my permanent store. She was about my age and a lot of fun and we worked very well together. She was pregnant and I had to play full General Manager while she was out on maternity leave, which was not fun for me. Quiznos was small, and it was easy to be the GM. Cosi was a much bigger operation with a lot more processes and paperwork and the only good that came from those three horrible months of my life is that I was given permission to open Monday through Friday because that's when we did the bulk of our business. My "assistant" was fresh out of training. I wasn't even compensated any extra for playing GM for several months, and I wasn't even asked if I wanted the job. At my initial meeting with Mike when I got back from Florida, he basically told me that's what would be happening, but I didn't feel like I had the option to request someone else step in. It wasn't like it was something I couldn't handle, but let's just say it's not something I would have wanted to do again, with that company anyway.

Over the course of the year after we got back, Eric and I continued to have problems. I missed Florida and wanted to go back, but he had hated the hot weather and the racism in the south, which I'll give him. Detroit is a very mixed city and we have a lot of black friends, and mixed couple friends with beautiful mixed babies, but Florida is a little behind the times and I hear it's much worse in other states. He didn't think he could get his job back at Sawgrass, which is the only way he'd go with me. He became very distant and nasty at times. We fought a lot. We broke up and got back together twice in one month. He finally got a call from Sawgrass saying he was welcome back at any time, so we did what we had done two years prior, sold most of what we had and moved down in his dad's minivan, and our two cars.

CHAPTER 8

This time we moved into an apartment in Ponte Vedra, that we really couldn't afford, which meant that his commute was only about five minutes and mine was about forty five minutes, but I was just glad to be back. We were paying just as much for a third the square feet and the worst layout I've ever lived in, which I didn't even realize was possible in a one bedroom apartment; but the grounds were beautiful, and the ocean was only a few blocks away. I could smell it from our balcony. Wayne had told me I could come back to Quiznos, but what he failed to mention was, it was just as a shift leader, there were no openings for a manager, and that meant a fair amount less money than I was expecting. His plan to supplement my income was to hire me as his little marketing wench for his smoked BBQ business that he was trying to get off the ground, but even after hours and hours of passing out fliers and telling people how delicious it was, without samples, no one wanted to order it, which was understandable. Problem was, we had agreed I'd be paid a percentage of every order that came in, and even 100% of zero is still zero.

When I learned that there was no management position available for me with Quiznos, I started interviewing with other restaurants. I knew my stuff, and by this point I knew how to interview and I was offered a management job with a Southern Mexican chain that hollers at you every time you walk in the door, but they were offering less than I wanted, I HATED the hours, and they couldn't promise me I wouldn't be put at the store on the opposite side of the city, which would be an hour commute, one way, so I turned it down. I also called every Panera Bread within the city to ask what the General Manager's name was so I could send a personalized cover letter with a resume in hopes they would pass it on to their District Manager. I got a call one Saturday morning from Kenny, the GM of the beaches Panera Bread only five minutes from our apartment asking if I could come in for an interview in an hour. I had narrowed down that if I was going to be stuck in the restaurant industry for a while, Panera Bread was the company I wanted to be with, hence the bombing of the resumes. They are a large corporate national chain and ever expanding that understands their managers are going to work more hours than they're scheduled, so they only schedule them for 45 hours, five days per week. I said absolutely and arrived five minutes early.

I thought the interview went great! He asked me about myself, what I was looking for in a company, obviously about my past work experiences, if I knew how to calculate food cost and balance a Profit and Loss statement, and then told me all about the company. If I hadn't been sold before, I definitely was after this interview, especially when I called several days later to follow up at 1:55pm and the girl that answered the phone thought he was still there and then came back to say he must have slipped out the back door. Cosi managers had to get to the store at the same time to open, 5am, but I never left before 5pm, and that was a good day. I wanted in. He had said he would pass on my information to the district manager and recommend me, but I never got a call.

The whole time Eric was back in Florida with me he was trying to get funding to go to turf school. He had decided he really loved being on the golf course, but in order to move up in course maintenance, you need a degree in turf management. He applied for several student loans, but just kept getting rejected as his credit was not stellar in those days.

The fighting at home continued. One day in early November Eric asked me if I was happy. He was being very vague and awkward, but he ultimately got to the point that he was glad that I was happy, but that he was not, and he was going to go back to Michigan and that I was welcome to come, but he understood if I didn't want to. I thought about it for a few days, but eventually I realized it was a long time coming and I gave him my blessing to go and try to find his happiness. He didn't leave for almost two months, which was difficult. We weren't really broken up because we were still sharing a bed, but we weren't really still together because we knew he was leaving. The real kicker is that everything was in my name because I'd had the better credit. The apartment lease, my car loan which still had four years left on it that I hadn't wanted to finance to begin with, a personal loan, a couple credit cards, a lot of bad financial decisions that I would like to have blamed on him, but I could have said no at any point. I had no idea how I was going to survive on what little I was making at Quiznos.

This is when I decided to become a stripper. I had a pole at home, had taken all of one pole dancing class, and knew I was pretty enough, and had a big ol' round booty for a short white girl that got me hit on all the time. I went to the one club in Jacksonville we had gone to before on our debaucherous night out with Mike in the beginning, and asked if they were hiring, to which the bouncer said they were always looking for dancers. I met with the manager, who asked me to show him my stomach to prove I didn't have stretch marks, and asked me to show him my tattoo, but didn't think it would be a problem. We decided my name should be "Susie" and that I would start the next night. The next day I went to work at Quiznos, borrowed a pair of shoes from the girlfriend of one of my coworkers, who was quite conveniently a dancer, and my shoe size, and stopped at an adult shop and bought a white outfit for my first night as everyone kept calling me "the virgin" to the stage.

My dad always had this policy of lurking in the shadows of a new situation. He had taught me to find a corner and observe until I felt comfortable, and this is what I intended to do for the first few nights. The few girls that I met were actually really nice and very helpful and wished me luck, not what I was expecting at all as I've known some other girls that have worked in the clubs and told me horror stories, so I'm guessing I just got lucky. One girl was sitting off to the side and invited me to sit with her, so I did, and a couple guys came over and sat with us. When it was my turn to go up I asked the DJ if he had any Halestorm, and he seemed surprised that I knew who they were, and I danced to the song "I get off." After that I even sold a dance to one of the guys that was sitting with us. As fate would have it though, the song that came on right as I was about to begin my dance was my song with Eric. You know how every couple has that one song that's "their song?" Well, ours came on, and somehow I got through the dance, but once it was over, I thanked the man and barely made it to the bathroom before I broke down sobbing, which several of the other girls saw. I was so embarrassed I told the manager I felt dirty and didn't think I could do it, to which he kindly asked me to tip out the DJ and security and that I could go. I still left with about fifty dollars, and that was after only three hours of not even trying, so I feel like had I stuck with it, I could have been taking home over five a night. But I also had this feeling I might come to loathe men altogether, and I didn't want that, so I just never went back, or to any other club like I had originally planned.

I called my dad in tears and told him the whole story because my dad and I could talk like that. I told him everything. He had already known Eric was about to leave, and he was still in Gainesville, Florida at this point, but he explained he'd been thinking about it, and how would I feel about him moving back to Jacksonville, and getting the three of us back in one house; him, me, and my brother, who was now staying with him since graduating. I liked this idea. I had always relied on the men in my life to take care of me, and this situation was no different. I wanted my dad to move back to Jacksonville and save me. This was the plan for a while.

My apartment had a very strict policy about breaking leases, but it turned out, they also now owned a complex on Southside with "studio" apartments that were hundreds of dollars a month cheaper, and I could transfer my lease over there for a minimal transfer fee. This would put me only twenty minutes from work, and I would have my own place, for the first time in my life. This terrified me. It was quite literally keeping me awake at night, the fear of living alone, and so I knew it was something I needed to do. And fortunately, I got promoted to Assistant Manager with Quiznos, so I got a raise, and was much closer to being able to support myself. My good friend, Rachel, was also looking to leave her job as the shot girl at a gay bar in Riverside, so she passed it off to me. This was another of my favorite jobs. I never felt like going because I had already worked all day, but every Friday night I would show up just before ten, the fabulous bartender would mix me a couple pitchers of brightly colored concoctions that I would pour into test tubes and sell for $2 each. The bar got one dollar, and I got one dollar, and I got to keep all my tips so I rarely left with less than $100 in four hours. This was enough that I could budget accordingly and make it through on my own.

I remember the day he left was Sunday, December 20, 2009, very early in the morning. I got up to see him off, but was so numb I didn't even cry. An hour later I went in and worked a full Sunday shift. It wasn't until I was getting off at about 3:00pm when Rachel and her friend, Nicky, came to visit me at work to see how I was doing that I just broke down. I wept like a baby in Rachel's arms. I really and truly believed that this was it and I would never see or hear from him again. I went to

Sneakers after work, but even that just made me miss him more because it was "our" bar, and everyone there was "our" friends, so I just went home and called Leah and cried to her for probably two hours before eventually falling asleep.

The next few days are kind of a blur, but I remember going to my Dad's for Christmas. My mother also drove down from Savannah and my dad's mother came up from her place in Leeseburgh, Florida, which is about an hour outside of Orlando. Christmas was a Friday this year and it was supposed to be my first night of work at the club, but thankfully my boss told me to enjoy my Christmas with my family. The plan was for my mother to follow me back to my apartment the next day, stay one night, and then leave the next morning to go back to Savannah. When she pulled a giant suitcase out of her trunk though, I learned that she was actually planning to stay the whole week and help me move into my studio the following weekend. I didn't have the heart to tell her I didn't need her, because honestly, I was still terrified of living alone.

I was aching inside from the loss of Eric's presence, and I did something rather stupid, but got very lucky, for lack of a better cliché. I had posted an ad on Craigslist in the "casual encounters" section. I had hundreds of responses, but the one I chose lived over in the Mayport area. We used fake names and emailed back and forth a few times before scheduling his place (because I didn't need some stranger knowing where I lived) the day after Christmas. I let Andrea know what I was doing, the address that I was going to, and that if I didn't call her within four hours to call the authorities in Jacksonville and send them to his house because I was probably dead or tied up in the basement, or likely elsewhere because Florida houses didn't have basements. Fortunately, I called her in less than four hours in tears because I didn't feel any better and I still missed Eric terribly. She was just glad I was still alive.

My dad and my brother came up on New Year's Eve to help me move into my studio across town. They got into a hit and run accident on the way though because apparently some scumbags were running from the police and broadsided my dad's Saturn running up onto the curb and then came back down in the street in front of him but he only caught the first three letters of the plate and I don't think they ever caught the guys. I remember he called to say they were going to be late and sounded so apologetic, and I was just glad they were okay! I really wouldn't have even needed him to help me move if it weren't for the couch and the dresser my mother wasn't strong enough to help me carry down the stairs.

At the new apartment, one of the neighbors came over to introduce herself while we were moving in. Her name was Carol and her little orange dog was Pumpkin. She was a very kind elderly woman and said if I ever needed anything, she was right in the next building over. I would see her from time to time and we would wave hello.

We spent the day moving and that night my dad, brother and I went to Sneakers to ring in the New Year: 2010. I remember what I posted to my Facebook status that night: "2009 was by far the most physically, mentally, emotionally and financially exhausting year of my life; so all I have to say to you 2010 is: bring it!"

This, was a colossal mistake.

CHAPTER 9

The hardest part of my breakup with Eric was looking at our now empty apartment the day I turned in my keys. I handed them over, barely made it out the door, and I broke down on the sidewalk, sobbing. In my moment of weakness, I texted him: "just tell me you miss me, and I'll never ask you for anything again." He wrote back immediately that of course he did and wanted to talk. My dad and mother were still in town for one more day so we agreed I would call him as soon as they had left. On January 2, 2010, at about two o'clock in the afternoon, I did.

We spent almost three hours on the phone that afternoon. He explained that leaving was simultaneously the worst and best decision he'd ever made. He had realized in the last two weeks that nothing in Detroit meant anything to him without his family (Apollo and me) there to share it with him. He admitted that he'd been a real asshole and had put a lot of really unfair stipulations on me, and that I was the only one that really knew him and understood him, and three hours boiled down into one sentence: he wanted to get married. Eventually, I agreed. We were going to wait a few years until we could afford a nice little ceremony, because we knew we weren't going to get any help from either of our families with that part, and I didn't have a ring or anything, and he was in Michigan and I in Florida with a brand new seven month lease that I was not about to break, but we were engaged.

The original plan was that once Eric got a job and saved up some money and found a reasonably priced place for us to live, that I would come back to Michigan. I had already emailed Mike, my District Manager at Cosi, and Lord knows why he said I was welcome back at any time, just let him know when I was coming. Well, he did say he was a little hesitant that I would leave again, but I had always done a good job while I was there and gave at least a month of notice before I left each time. However, no matter how diligently he looked, Eric could not find a decent job. He had sold his car in Florida to have money to go back to Michigan on, but his position had been filled at the independent dealer, and the Saturn he had worked at for the year in between had closed down, obviously, when Saturn went out of business. He was crashing on a friend's couch and borrowing his dad's minivan he wasn't using at the time, and he was running out of money quickly.

Meanwhile, in Florida, I was actually loving living alone. It wasn't terrifying like I thought it would be. I had my very own place for the first time, and it was mine. I took pride in keeping it neat, organized and clean. I thought that I would be bored and lonely, but I wasn't. I was working so much at Quiznos, and Fridays at the Club, and Eric called me every day, and if it wasn't him then it was Andrea, or I was at Sneakers with Jamie and the crew, or over at my Dad's, who was now back in Jacksonville. Aside from my fiancé living eleven hundred miles away from me, this was a good time in my life. I proved to myself, even though it was for only three short months, that I could live alone and self-sustain, and it was very empowering. It taught me I didn't need a man to save me when things got tough.

At the end of March though, Eric realized he was not going to find a decent job in Michigan and decided to come back to Florida and stay with me. He hated Jacksonville, but we settled on Tampa which was a much bigger city with sports teams, which is very important to him (yes, Jacksonville has the jaguars, but let's be honest, they're an expansion team that had only been there eleven years at the time, and they still can't sell out a game because just about everyone in Jacksonville is from somewhere else). It's very much like a really big small town. It was the largest city in the country by actual land mass, and most things are very far apart from one another, but the people have a very small town way about them, or at least the natives, which are few and far between in most of the areas we frequented with the rest of the other transplants. Eric always worked blue collar jobs though, and those were usually heavy with natives because as far as I could tell at the time, the only industry in Jacksonville is insurance and the navy. I've never much loved working in restaurants, but I didn't mind it nearly as much in Florida because it was sunny and warm damned near every day. I was perfectly fine with the idea of moving to Tampa.

I knew this wasn't going to happen by early May though. Every year the PGA Tour holds a golf tournament called "The Players" at TPC Sawgrass, usually on Mother's Day weekend. We had gone the first year we were there because Eric got free passes as a groundskeeper of the course. The second year we were there he still had friends working there and they gave him a couple of their passes. I don't remember why he initially hadn't wanted to go back to Sawgrass when he came back in March, but he was working at a much lower-end course over in the Orange Park area at the time. At the tournament though he ran into some old co-workers that told him some news about some changes happening or something, and that night he suggested putting off moving to Tampa another year because he was thinking of going back to Sawgrass and didn't want to be that guy that just kept coming and going (the way I had been with Cosi, but I don't think this is what he was getting at). I just knew right then we were never going to make it to Tampa.

Then, a few weeks later, I was checking the history in my browser on my computer, and discovered that he'd been looking at apartments in Chicago. When I asked him about it, he had to tell me he was thinking maybe we should move there. I assume most of you have seen the movie *Apollo 13* with Tom Hanks among other greats, and he has this line about a third of the way into the movie: "fellas, we just lost the moon." This is how I felt. I thought Tampa was a fabulous compromise and Tampa was my moon. Or any other city in Florida, where it was warm and sunny and beautiful and close to my dad. Nothing against Chicago, it's a toddling town according to Ol' Blue Eyes; I've been there several times, it's wonderful, but it might as well just be Detroit for how far it is from Florida, and it's way more expensive, and there was no way that Eric was going to walk Apollo all winter like he kept promising me. This was the plan for maybe a month or so, but as the end of our lease got closer and we still had no savings, we put that off too. Thankfully.

I never particularly liked living on the ground floor. My patio faced the parking lot, was right up against the sidewalk so anyone walking by could see my entire apartment if I didn't keep the blinds closed, and anyone walking behind the building could see into my bedroom if the blinds weren't closed, so it kind of felt like a shoebox. Fortunately, there was an upstairs unit opening up that would be available at the end of our lease for the same amount. I don't think Eric wanted to move units, but he said if I really wanted to then we could. I was surprised. Eric was usually kind of a my way or the highway kind of guy and I was just sort of used to not getting my way somewhat more often than not because very few things were important enough to me to argue over, so I would just concede; but I remember feeling even more in love with him after he pretty much single handedly moved us into the upstairs unit in the next building over, simply because I wanted to. It had a private balcony, a much better view out the back window, and even a garbage disposal and a dishwasher, which the previous unit didn't have because it was handicapped accessible so everything was designed to roll a wheel chair underneath.

Upon moving though, we obviously had to sign another lease, so I knew I had at least seven more months in Florida. A few weeks after the move I got it into my head that I was going to check with Panera Bread again, and just let them know I was still interested, so I sent Kenny an email one morning, from Quiznos, and got a call on my cell phone only a few hours later from Steve Lisner, the Jacksonville District Manager. We scheduled an interview at the San Jose store for several days later.

He apologized for not contacting me sooner, but was glad I'd followed up because they were indeed looking to hire more managers at that time as they would be opening another store in St. Augustine in just a few months. I think he liked that I was honest and admitted that I didn't absolutely love working in restaurants, but it was a stable salary, and art and music didn't pay the rent. He had wanted to write the great American novel out of college and started working in a restaurant so he could at least feed himself and just worked his way up. We talked about writing and music and somehow we got on the topic of vitamins, and very little about the company, but I imagine Kenny had already let him know that I would be a decent manager and he was just trying to get a feel for my personality, which of course, is "sparkling." I thought this interview went just as well as the first and several days later he called me while I was walking Apollo and offered me exactly what I had planned on asking for, which is more than I would have taken but left me bargaining room. We agreed I would start training in just over two weeks at the Bartram Park store, which was only about fifteen minutes from my apartment.

The first three days of training were actually Baker Training, which takes place over night. I had to show up at 10pm and work until 6am, which really threw off my circadian rhythm for a few days, but then I was given the weekend off to catch up. I loved Panera. I loved that all the bread was baked fresh every day and whatever wasn't sold at closing time was donated to local charities instead of being thrown away. I loved the extra security measures that were strictly adhered to of not even opening the back door after dark because all of my previous restaurants had been robbed that way. I loved that they had an armored car service come pick up the deposits from the store as opposed to sending the manager to the bank, as there were always stories of people getting shot and killed over a day's deposit. I loved the benefits, the schedule, the people, the two weeks of vacation my first year and that there were stores all over the place if we needed to borrow anything, which everyone needed to do from time to time. If Eric hadn't taken my new position with my significant raise as an excuse to quit his job at the low-end golf course (which, to be fair, was mistreating him grossly and very poorly run), this would have been a lucrative time in my life. It was, at least, a generally happy time.

Sunday September 26, 2010 around 9pm or so, cop cars and a fire truck came screaming into our parking lot. Carol's daughter, who came to visit her pretty frequently, was there. They knocked several times, but I guess she didn't answer because they broke the door down and a second later her daughter screamed "NOOO" in the most horrific, strained, painful scream I think I've ever heard. To this day I can still remember the sound of her finding her mother, dead. I cried. I continued to cry for the rest of the night. Not because I had known Carol all that well, but because I was so afraid of the first time I would lose someone close to me, like my dad. Eric had lost his mother to cancer about nine years before and I asked him a lot of questions and he was a real comfort, but I just remember that being my biggest fear in life for years because I knew it was inevitable.

CHAPTER 10

The next day, Monday September 27, 2010, I was closing. It was my last week of training and Laurie, my training assistant manager told me to go have a cigarette before dinner rush started. I never keep my phone on me at work, always in my purse in the office, but would check it on the occasional break, and this particular night there was a message from my grandmother that my dad had gone to the hospital after a fainting spell he'd had at work. He didn't want me to know, but if you know my grandmother, no one tells her what to do and I am glad she called me. I called my brother, who had his phone off, and then called my dad, and his was still on and learned that he had passed out in the lawn on Thursday, drove himself and Tom home later that day, somehow coached Tom (who had never learned to drive a car, just practiced a couple times here and there) how to drive them back to work on Friday, but wasn't able to concentrate or get any work done, and they went back home. His policy was always to sleep it off, and never go to a doctor. When he didn't feel better by Monday, he tried going to an urgent care clinic, but those are for minor illness and accidents and they told him he needed a hospital. He eventually made it to the hospital by the beach around 5pm; about the same time my grandmother had called me.

I ran back inside, told Laurie what happened and she told me to go, even helped me figure out where the hospital was and how to get there. It was a good thing I did go because not too long after I got there, they determined that they needed to move my dad to the main hospital downtown; that he had to go in an ambulance, and Tom could not ride in the ambulance, so he would have been stuck at the hospital.

We stopped by their house to get my dad his phone charger, electronic cigarette, toothbrush and glasses and hurried to the main hospital, but it was too late in the night to do anything that day as all of the doctors and techs had gone home. We stayed for a little while, but then I took Tom home, and went home to Eric. All we knew so far was that my dad had a brain tumor, but we didn't know if it was malignant, or operable, or fatal; simply that it was there.

Fortunately, I was off the next day, picked Tom up and we went straight to the hospital. They took his vitals every few hours, did another MRI and a CT scan, did his EKG twice because they couldn't believe his lungs were so clear after smoking two to three packs a day for the last forty-five years. They scheduled his biopsy for Thursday morning. His surgeon, Dr. Chandler, was a super nice guy, and very informative. I liked him and I trusted him. He really made me believe he had my dad's best interest in mind. It took about four hours, but Eric came to the hospital with us that day and I don't know what Tom did, but Eric and I walked around. We went down by the river and saw a few dolphins swimming, which was not uncommon in the Jacksonville River. Fortunately, the operation was a success and you couldn't even see the scar and they didn't even have to shave any of his hair. We wouldn't have lab results back for a few days though.

I decided to go to work Friday because I couldn't just keep sitting in the hospital room unable to help the situation, and Panera had been gracious enough already letting me leave in the middle of my shift on Monday night and giving me an extra day off to be there for the biopsy. Tom had figured out a bus route he could take to get to the hospital and back, so I wasn't really needed. I told everyone at work what was going on that hadn't already heard.

Saturday morning, October 2, 2010, the surgeon pulled my brother and I aside into a consultation room at the end of the hall to let us know the results had come back late the night before. It was a Glioblastoma Multiforme, which is a very aggressive malignant tumor, a stage four, the fastest growing, and he had about a month to live. I remember thinking his birthday was in exactly one month. What if he didn't even make it until his birthday?

I kept it together while we all went back to my dad's room and the surgeon told him the news. My dad seemed somewhat un-phased by this information, but I think he already knew. If there was ever a man I knew that was more in tune with his own body than the rest of the world, it was my dad. He ate processed garbage, smoked, and drank in moderation, but he was also very into martial arts, yoga, meditation, and he had read lots of books about a lot of things, and a bunch of those were about the body and mind. He admitted to me later he'd already noticed himself "getting stupid" for over a month leading up to the fainting spell, which was later determined to have likely been a mini seizure. He just hadn't gone to a doctor because he didn't have health insurance, hated doctors, and figured it was likely something critical that he didn't have the money to fix.

As part of my dad moving back to Jacksonville, he had agreed to go back to work for his previous boss from his previous company that had gone under. He was working on a new online gaming program and needed my dad's programming expertise and my brother came as a bonus because he could test the games and let them know where the bugs were. Problem with this scenario is they were paid with promises of certain salaries once said program actually got a buyer, which of course, it never did. They were working for him for months, essentially for free. My dad had gone to him a month or two prior and told him he needed at least a minimum to keep stringing them along, but that was only enough for rent, utilities, gas, groceries, the bare essentials. I had told him before he took the job that I didn't like the idea, and get something in writing about what they would get if the project never went anywhere, but he didn't, and they got nothing. I feel like if my dad had a real job, with health insurance, he might have gone and gotten checked out sooner, and he may have chosen to fight it. But he didn't.

My dad was always the smart one in the room, and he knew it and he was proud of it. He said he could already tell the difference in the way his thoughts were processing, and he didn't think he'd ever get that back, and he didn't want to live as a "stupid person" and decided not to proceed with treatment, he was just going to let it happen. He also believed it would be only a month. He entered hospice care almost immediately. The administrative nurse that came to his house to enroll him, Mary, was very kind and had pretty long red hair. My dad liked her. She initially admitted him at a fifty percent capacity because he taken a bad turn since getting home from the hospital. He was having a very difficult time using the restroom, and the hospice people ultimately determined he had a urinary tract infection and would need a catheter for the rest of his life. The toxins in his urine were pretty much poisoning his body, but once he was finally able to excrete them, he seemed like he was doing much better.

I started going over every other day, running errands for them, doing grocery shopping, picking up whatever they needed. I remember about a week after the diagnosis, I drove by a wedding dress shop on A1A, and I broke down in tears, which was common these days. I was never the girl that dreamed of her wedding. I was terrified of marriage, and probably never would have gotten up the balls to walk down the aisle if my dad hadn't gotten sick. The only thing that ever mattered to me about my wedding was that my daddy walk me down the aisle. I called Eric in tears because my daddy wasn't going to be around to walk me down the aisle, and he said "well, then let's get married now." I don't know why this hadn't occurred to me, but like I said, I didn't need some big ceremony, I wasn't religious, I actually got really excited by how simple we kept everything. We went to the courthouse on Wednesday to get the marriage license, set up that the magistrate lady would come to my dad's house around 6pm on Saturday, I went to a thrift store and picked out a cute white sundress for all of six dollars, and baked us a cake.

I even worked the day of my wedding, October 16th, which also turned out to be Sweetest Day, but a lot of states don't even know what that is. I was scheduled until 5pm. Everyone knew I was getting married that evening though so they kicked me out around 4pm. I rushed home, showered, did my makeup, brought my dress, shoes, and the dollar store veil and flower bouquet I had made and drove over to my dad's, where Eric was already waiting. I called before I got there and he waited out in the back yard until the magistrate got there, and I was ready, so he wouldn't see me on the day of the wedding. It was magical, in our own little way. My uncle Pat, great uncle Bill, and my mother were all there because they were already in town to see my dad. The only thing I would change is that I wish Eric's dad, Norm and his wife, Karen, could have made it down, but they weren't able to. That, and I wish we had brought Apollo.

My mother wore the dress she had brought in case there was a funeral, which was off white with angels and very pretty, but I knew she had brought it for a funeral, not for a wedding. She attended the ceremony portion, but shortly after the "I dos," she went inside and went to sleep, which honestly was probably better, because the rest of us proceeded to get rather intoxicated, like everyone should do at a wedding!

My dad's own mother however, didn't make it down to Florida until November 8th. I could probably write a whole other book about her, but let's just say she doesn't handle death well. She lost her father at a young age, and hasn't gone to many funerals since, even though she's lost a sister, a sister-in-law, a lot of friends, a son, and a husband. I think she only went to her husband's service because she had put it together, it was expected. I imagine if she could have gotten out of it, she would have. She had a Florida house she went to every year around early November and could not make it down before then for lots of perfectly good reasons. Thankfully, my dad was still doing okay when she finally made it, five weeks after he was given one month.

She came up every few weeks and my dad started calling her every night. After my grandmother visited the first time, my dad asked my mother to move in to their house to be his full time caregiver, as she was not working at the time, and I don't think he wanted to put that much pressure on Tom, who was very good at keeping track of what medicine he was supposed to take and when, and cooking, but he never wanted to go outside, he wasn't very good at cleaning anything, and frankly, I don't know why. I think, honestly, that it was because he wanted them to re-strengthen their bond because Tom was going to have nowhere to go once my dad wasn't around to take care of him.

This only lasted about a month though. She was always spouting her bible verses, and wanting to pray, and making it known she felt like she was in "enemy territory" and as my dad descended he became very short tempered. He was ready to go and had stopped eating or drinking anything with calories. He drank only water or black coffee, and even asked his nurses if any of his medicines or vitamins had any calories. My uncle was gracious enough to be sending him money to pay his rent and bills, and he qualified for food stamps, which Tom used to cook meals for himself and anyone else who was visiting. I wasn't there for any of the real blowouts, but I guess it eventually got so bad that my dad told her to leave and Tom called the cops when she wouldn't. She moved back home to Savannah the next day and visited every so often.

I was still visiting every other day and watching him slowly descend into a clumsy, constantly confused, angry retarded zombie. The location of the tumor in his brain was affecting his speech and he would frequently not be able to find the right words for things and it was always a process to figure out what he was trying to say, which just made him frustrated. It was also a real eye-opener that he couldn't even dial a phone because he would say "five" and point to the nine, or any other number, so he needed someone with him at all times. Panera had been very supportive of my situation and kept me at my training store where I already knew everyone, and was only scheduling me mid-shifts so there was always another manager present in case I needed to leave at any point. But then the St. Augustine store opened and they had to move me and a few other people around, which was fine, but it was still going to be a big shock to go to a new store and learn a whole new team of people. My dad had also not eaten in over a month, and Eric was still not working, almost four months now since he had quit the golf course.

Needless to say, I was in a very low place. I had borrowed my mother's set of Dave Ramsey cd's that I had been listening to in the car in my many miles I was driving between home, work, and my dad's. Dave Ramsey, if you don't know, is a relatively well known financial planning guru with lots of neat little tips and tricks to getting out of debt, staying out, and building a nest egg to pass down and basically "change your family tree." He's very funny and interesting though, and also a man of faith, which he actually leaves out of his lectures, which I appreciated and the reason I actually made it through the whole series. The last disc in the series though was the story of Christ, and how much he loves every one of us, and how the angels in heaven would just have a royal party if I accepted him into my heart. So I did. I figured, hell, what could it hurt? Everything was turning to grits around me anyways. And Dave made a very convincing argument. So I repeated the words, out loud, in my car on my way home on December 20th. I didn't hear any trumpets or celebrating, but I felt like a weight had been lifted. When I got home, Eric informed me he had an interview with BMW in Detroit in two days. He had also already spoken to his father and turned out he was leaving his Florida house the next day to drive back to Detroit and said he could hitch a ride if we met him at the freeway exit, and I just so happened to be off the next day. This may have been just a coincidence, but it was still a big one.

What also may have been an even bigger coincidence is that a few days later, my brother randomly checked my dad's bank account which he wasn't even using anymore because it was nearly empty, and there had been a direct deposit of Social Security we didn't know was coming. The hospice social worker had apparently taken care of everything, and he would be receiving almost enough once a month to float him, so he wouldn't have to continue living off his brother, which I know he hated. He took twenty-four hours to think about it, but ultimately decided to start eating again. I was so happy I cried for an hour.

What was probably also another coincidence is that my dad had also insisted on starting to divvy out who was going to get what of his things, and since Tom didn't drive, it was determined Eric and I would get the car. It wasn't worth much since the accident, but it was still plenty drivable, so we decided to sell Eric's Honda Civic to buy him a new set of mechanic's tools and box to keep them in, which are very expensive. The day of his interview in Detroit, I listed and sold his car in Florida, for the exact price he found a box with complete set of tools listed for on Craigslist in Detroit.

The following morning I had my transition day to my

new store, which turned out to be the San Jose location, where I'd had my interview with Steve, where I had done my baker training, and coincidentally, where Kenny was now, who I'd had my initial interview with, so it wasn't nearly as big of a shock. It was only a few minutes farther from my house, and had a younger, more fun staff; probably because the management was too lenient on them. I had just found out Eric got the job in Detroit, so I knew I'd be transferring in a few months, so I wasn't about to rock the boat and have everyone hate me being the brand new manager that was then going to up and leave.

I had always known Eric wanted to be in Detroit, and in my grief early on in my dad's illness I told him that once my father passed, if he wanted to go back, we could. Eric had spent the last few months at home studying for hours at a time to take his ASE certification tests to become a nationally certified mechanic and he passed two of them. He only needed one to become employed, but planned to take the others in the near future. I didn't realize it would happen so quickly, but it was only several days after he got his test results that he found the BMW job posting, called to set up the interview, and clearly nailed it. They wanted him to start Monday, January 2nd. This gave him just enough time to fly back on Christmas Eve, spend a few days with me and my family, pack as much of his stuff as he could into the now-his Saturn, and drive back.

Yet another coincidence that happened this week is Andrea's roommate had recently moved out and she was looking for someone else to rent out her spare bedroom. She offered it to Eric for very cheap so that he'd have somewhere to stay and could save some money for when I made it up, because our initial plan was that I would stay until my dad passed. Funny thing was, my dad wanted to move back to Detroit too. In the beginning he was okay with the fact that he was going to die. He was welcoming of it. Several months in now though, the tumor was doing a real number on his brain, and the hospice people had told us to expect certain things, one of which was denial. He was convinced he was going to reconnect with Mike, his former Tai-Chi teacher, and he would heal him. He wanted to get another dog. He insisted his house have a fenced yard so that he could get another dog.

This conversation with the rest of the family did not go very well. My grandmother absolutely hated the idea, and she made it known. Maybe Tom and I were in denial too, but he had made it several months now and was still able to walk, shower, feed himself and whatnot, he just had some neurological issues sometimes, but he seemed like he might keep going up to another year. We cleared it with his hospice doctors and had him all set up to transfer into Michigan Hospice once we got there. This was probably not the best idea, but he really wanted to go. I think deep down he just didn't want to keep me from my husband, but we'd been apart for months at a time before and understood this is probably what was going to happen again, but he wouldn't hear it. He insisted on moving back to the Detroit area at the end of February when his lease was up.

I looked at quite a few housing options on Craigslist, and most of them seemed to be offered by one guy, so I called his people and tried to schedule an appointment for the Saturday I would be in town, about three weeks before our move date. The agent I spoke to just told me to call back once I actually was in town. I called him from the airport the Friday I landed, and left a message that I would be expecting to meet with him the next morning to go look at a couple houses I was interested in. I called him about 10:30am after Eric and I had gotten some breakfast and had to re-explain to this man who I was and why I was calling, and remind him I only had this one day to look at houses because I was flying out tomorrow. I think he was in the middle of something, but he met us at one of the houses about an hour later. This one did not have a fenced yard and was kind of a shithole, pardon my potty mouth, but this is what my dad could afford. I knew it would be cleaned up before he moved in. The man also showed us another property, but there were stairs to get up to the front door, and stairs to get up to the bedroom, and I knew that wouldn't work very well as he was already needing help walking. This man showing us places had to get to another appointment, but he took all of my information and criteria and sent me a list of about ten properties that roughly matched. I forwarded them to Tom and let him decide, but I was already back in Florida by this point and everything else was processed through phone calls and emails. I never saw the house he chose.

On my flight out of Detroit Monday night, about twenty minutes into the air, the flight attendants went running to the back of the plane. One came on the loudspeaker and asked if there was a doctor on board. There was a nurse. Apparently, a man had suffered a heart attack, and this nurse had likely saved his life, and we emergency landed in Cincinnati so that he could be rushed to a hospital. I was already fighting back tears, and the young woman I was sitting next to and I became very close for the next hour before we were finally allowed to take back off. Needless to say, none of us made our connections, which were all the last flights out for the evening, but the airline was kind enough to put us up at a local hotel for the night with vouchers for food from the airport for breakfast, and we were all booked on the first flight out to our final destinations. Fortunately, I didn't have to work until 2pm the next day, so I had enough time to fly in at 11am, go back by dad's and pick up Apollo before running home for a shower. Overall, this whole trip just felt unsuccessful, aside from the fact I got to see my husband for the first time in almost two months.

My dad was doing pretty well in January, but by February, I started to wonder if he was going to make it to the move. We already knew the house they were going to be moving into was fully carpeted, but he got very upset when Tom was about to throw out a rug they wouldn't need. He screamed and yelled and just kept saying "but it's my stuff!" For the first time he looked at me like he didn't know who I was, and then the same to Tom, and then just started screaming "Die! Die! Die!" Which was his way of saying he was ready to die. Then he started crying, which I had never seen him do. This sort of thing was happening more and more and he was losing the use of his limbs. He could no longer hold up his own weight and needed help in and out of a wheelchair by the week of the move.

We had all previously decided the easiest way to move everyone back up to Detroit was for my dad to fly up with my brother a couple days prior, and Eric would fly back down from Michigan to help me pack up the shared moving truck, which he would drive back, and I would drive my car with Apollo. This would allow me time to clean both their house, and our apartment without distraction and get us both our deposits back. The day that they flew out, Thursday, February 25, 2010, was probably the longest, most stressful, and exhausting day of my life.

I got to their house about 7:45am and it took both Tom and I to get my dad into the car, who was pretty confused all the time by this point, which had only come on several days prior. We put their bags in the trunk and I drove them to the airport. A very nice man who worked for the airport helped my dad into a wheelchair and told Tom where to go to check in for their flight. I went to a local coffee and donut shop to wait for Tom to call me that they had successfully made it through security and were waiting at their gate before heading back to their house to finish their packing, and clean their house. Their flight left at about 10am, they had a connection in Atlanta, and didn't land in Detroit until about 5pm. I was terrified all day that something was going to go wrong on the plane; but thankfully, that part was smooth. Tom called to let me know they landed safely, Dad was okay, and our Uncle was there to pick them up and take them to their new house. I was about done at their place so I went back home to shower before driving to the Orlando airport to pick up Eric, who was flying in that night.

While I was in the shower I got a call from Tom, in hysterics. Apparently, the house they had chosen was a complete mess, was ridiculously cold with the only heating vent in the living room, there was no overhead lighting in any room but the kitchen, and Tom had said something rather rude and ungrateful to our uncle and he left. My dad was rocking back and forth on a chair repeating "so cold. So cold." Tom had done a good job of taking care of our dad in Florida where there were nurses he could call, and me to drive them around, but now he was eleven hundred miles away with no car, and it was February in Michigan and he didn't have any idea where he was, or anything else for that matter, and he couldn't leave my dad alone. I felt so helpless.

I called the only people I knew would do whatever they could to help me, the Miltons. They were the parents of my ex-boyfriend that I had always kept in touch with and considered my second family. I called them "mommy-almost, and daddy-almost" and they called me "daughter-almost" and they are probably the kindest people I've ever known. I think they were at Costco when I called, but they could tell from my voice that it was an emergency and they dropped what they were doing to go get my dad and Tom and take them to a nearby hotel.

I called the landlord, who was clearly at some casino somewhere because I could hear the machines in the background once he finally answered and I explained they could not stay in that house. When he insinuated that I had seen the house, I further explained to him that was my intention, but his man had treated me like I was unimportant and didn't make time for me when I was in town, even though I had called him twice the week before he was to show me the properties; which I think was news to him. Fortunately, he had another house only a few miles away that was still a dump, but at least it had heating vents in every room, which you would think every house in Michigan should have, but apparently not. It also had a fenced yard, and a garage, neither of which they needed, but the rent was only ten dollars more.

While I was making these phone calls however, I was drying off from my half a shower, getting dressed, walking Apollo and getting back in my car to go pick up Eric from the Orlando airport. If you're wondering why Eric didn't just fly into the Jacksonville airport, it's because there are very few direct flights from DTW to JAX and they were all quite a bit more money than we wanted to spend, and he didn't want to take more than Friday and Monday off, so he had to be able to work a full day Thursday and fly out at 9pm or so, direct. We found a cheap flight that went straight to Orlando, which was just over two hours away.

Halfway through my drive to Orlando, just after the Miltons called me to let me know my dad and Tom were safely at their hotel for now, traffic stopped. The entire freeway of I-95 slowly came to a complete stop and didn't move for probably twenty minutes or more. There had apparently been a very bad accident just up ahead and they closed the whole freeway and were re-routing traffic across the median and back up the opposite way to a detour connection. At that moment, I thanked God that the house shenanigans had made me several minutes late from my desired departure time.

I called Eric and left him a message that I would likely be late because of the accident and the detour and whatnot, but not to panic because I was on my way and would be there as soon as I could. His plane was a little delayed and I ended up making better time than expected, so he didn't have to wait long. We finally made it back home about 2:30 in the morning.

The next morning we went to pick up the moving truck, as soon as they opened at 8:00am. This was a very long day of packing up my dad's house, driving back to our apartment to pack up our stuff, then going back to my dad's for the carpet cleaners, and the final walk through with his landlords while Eric finished packing our apartment into the truck. That night we ate pizza off paper towels and played cards on the floor and tried to enjoy each other's company though we'd bickered all day.

We bickered quite a bit the next day too. The whole weekend really. I was just heartbroken to be leaving Florida. The time before I knew I'd be visiting, and maybe we'd move back, but for some reason, I just knew that this time, that was it. I didn't have any family there anymore and only a few friends left at this point, and Eric had no interest in ever going back, so I just knew that I wouldn't have much reason to go either. I resented him for this, even though it was not his fault. I resented my brother for having no job and being able to be my dad's full time caregiver while I had to work. I even resented my dad for refusing to fight his cancer. There was a lot of anger inside me and I took it out on Eric while we were driving back. If I had to psychoanalyze myself, that would be my quasi professional opinion; but what do I know?

CHAPTER 11

When we got back to Michigan, Eric showed me around the house he had picked out for us, which took about 4.2 seconds as I'm pretty sure it was smaller than our apartment we'd had in Florida which was $260/month less, but at least this place had a small fenced yard and a one car garage we never parked in. We unloaded our stuff into our house and then drove the two miles to my dad's new house and my uncle helped unload my dad's and Tom's stuff before going to pick them up from their hotel. This place was much more to their liking, even though it had yellow walls and purple carpet, but they didn't seem to mind. I took pictures of how dirty and cluttered with debris the place was for future reference, but did not put up a stink to the landlord as I suspected I was already the newest pebble in his shoe, and that is not like me.

Once I knew they were settling in and going to be okay for a couple days I went back home to my own new house in shambles. Fortunately, I had just hit my six months anniversary with Panera so I was allowed to use one of my vacation weeks to move and not take unpaid time off, but I only had two more days off at this point and I wanted to get my house in some sort of unpacked order before returning to work at my new store, which was about thirty minutes from my new house. One of those days off I did drive out to the new store and met my new District Manager, Chris, and General Manager, Sherry, both of whom seemed nice enough to work with; but I'd never met anyone working for Panera that I didn't get along with, yet.

It was a bit of a rocky start at the Bloomfield Hills store, I still felt brand new to the company as my dad had gotten sick right at the end of my training, and no one expected me to do much or learn much while he was dying. I wanted to learn, but I was the extra manager in my training store, and then basically became the closing bitch, at my temporary store in Jacksonville. Kenny had started showing me inventory, but once they all knew I was transferring, I think they didn't feel like wasting any more training hours on me and decided to let the Michigan stores teach me what else I needed to know. I remember Sherry told me once "just let me know what you don't know and I can teach you;" which I found rather laughable, because to me, it was obvious that I wouldn't know what it was that I didn't know and needed to be taught, but I got through it.

I'm not proud to say it, but I think I only went over to see my dad once or twice over the next couple weeks. I had all kinds of perfectly rational excuses in my mind, but I'm pretty sure I knew he was close to going, and I wasn't ready. He was getting really bad. Confined to a hospital bed they had brought in and mostly paralyzed. My brother and I had to change his diapers in his last few days. The hospice nurses would come by the house every morning to give him a sponge bath, and to check on my brother, who wasn't eating. One of the nurses even brought him lunch one time. I do remember in his last couple days, once he had stopped responding, they put him on morphine, which had to be administered every four hours. I offered to come by and stay the night Friday March 11, 2011, so Tom could get a full night's rest. I remember trying to sleep in my dad's recliner, in the living room with his hospital bed, and I couldn't get that David Bowie song out of my head, "Space

Oddity" which my dad had often sung, because his name was Tom. I kept reciting the part where he sings "this is Major Tom to ground control, I'm stepping through the door, and I'm floating in the most peculiar way, and the stars look very different today." I don't think I slept at all that night.

The next morning, once my brother had woken I told him I was going home for a shower, running some errands and I would be back later that night, after dinner time. Around 5pm he called me and said that I should probably hurry back because dad's breathing had changed and he suspected it could be soon. I had just finished making dinner and told him I'd be over as soon as I was done eating, but he called back about a half hour later and I could hear in his voice that he did not want to be alone so I rushed over. I remember crying in my car and begging God to just take him, that I was ready. That I didn't want him to suffer anymore and if he was keeping him on earth for me to please just take him, I would be okay.

When I got to the house, about 5:45pm, it was pretty clear he had passed, and I wasn't there when he'd gone. Tom was still sitting at the side of his bed, holding his hand, and wasn't sure if he was truly gone because the bed the hospice people had loaned him constantly filled and deflated with air and it sounded like he may have been breathing, but he wasn't. The most recent morphine pill was still between his gum and his lip, undissolved, and Tom had given it to him at 4pm. His eyes were half open and were just, lifeless. This is when I learned that the movies lie, and you cannot close someone's eyes that has just died, they will just pop back open.

The rest of the evening is a bit of a blur, but I know I called Eric, and then our uncle, and then Sherry at work, and then my mother, who didn't answer. Our uncle came over and called their mother while Tom and I called the hospice people and they came and checked all of his medicines back in. We then called the funeral home we had decided to go with and two men showed up with a van and a gurney and suggested that maybe we go for a walk because it can be very traumatizing for family to see a loved one get zipped up and taken away, so we did just that. We walked down to the end of the block and turned around just in time to see them wheeling him out and into the van. We both turned back around immediately, but they were right. My dad was in that bag on that gurney going into that van to be cremated, and he was never coming back. The only thing that brought me comfort in this moment is that they had let me pack him a bag that would be cremated with him. I used his favorite beach bag and packed it with his swimsuit, a towel, a pack of cigarettes and a couple books I knew he liked. Who knows if they really burned it with him, but I'm glad they humored me if not.

All of this obviously took several hours. Once everything was situated, all the important people were notified, and I checked that Tom was going to be alright, I went back home. I always felt bad about that, leaving him alone in the house our father had just died in. I should have invited him to come stay with us for the night or a few days. Even if he didn't take me up on it, I should have offered, but I didn't. Instead I went home to Eric and we went to our local watering hole, Danny's, and a bunch of our friends met us and I proceeded to get drunk. I got the kind of drunk that I never get because I don't like not being in control of my situation. Not since I was thirteen and I woke up in the closet have I been drunker than I was that night. Eric was driving. My father, my rock, my best friend in the world had just died. Even though I knew it was coming, and had almost six months to prepare, the books were right. It hurt like a motherfucker. Needless to say, I don't remember much of this night. One thing I do remember is what I posted as my Facebook status that night:

"Kids, gone to the beach. –Dad"

The next day I realized my mother had never called me back. I had called her personal phone and her work cell phone as she was currently working as a hospice secretary, go figure, and left similar messages on both, but she never called. So around 11am on Sunday, I called her again. She was at church. Service had just let out, but no, she hadn't received either of my messages. I told her she should probably sit down and then that dad had died the night before. She wailed. I don't know if I should have told her to go home and then call me back, but she would have just insisted I tell her. I just pictured her sitting on some bench in the church lobby on the phone, sobbing, and everyone walking by her wondering what was so horrible. I felt bad about that too, but I don't know what else I should have done.

Over the course of that next day I scheduled his service for the coming Wednesday, and informed everyone I could think of that might want to attend, and posted the information to the blog I had started for him back when he was diagnosed. I also went to the funeral home to sign some paperwork and select his urn. There was one I thought he would love. It was just a solid golden rectangular cube, but it was very geometrical and it reminded me of one of his favorite mathematical principles: the golden rectangle. The only piece of artwork he had ever made was a poster-sized collage of colorful felt squares that demonstrated the golden rectangle principle, and I had sewn him a fleece blanket many years later for a father's day present in the same vein.

We were blessed with a beautiful day the afternoon of his service, even though it was March in Michigan. I like to think he helped with that. He had never even wanted a service, but understood that they are really for the remaining living for closure, so gave me permission to throw him one if I wanted. We didn't have any music, or any real format, and he wasn't a religious man so there was no clergy or anything, but a lot of friends and family showed up. A whole bunch of people I hadn't seen in years, and honestly, I don't think he had seen in years, from his old days with Compuware, came and told stories of him that I had never heard. That was my favorite part. My friend, Rachel, whom I hadn't seen or spoken to in probably fifteen years came and told stories of how she remembered my dad. Rob Fender, one of my best friends growing up, also gave a great speech about how powerful cancer must be, because he never thought anything could kill Tom Barry. Neither did I.

The next day I had to take my mother, who had flown in for the service, back to the airport. Once she released me from her hug and walked inside, I left. I felt the most overwhelming sense of emptiness. This was the first moment since my father had passed, really since he had been diagnosed, that I had nothing to do. I've always been good at keeping myself busy at whatever task I was taking care of. For the past six months I was learning a new job, taking care of my father, getting married, planning a move for two households, moving, learning a new store, planning a funeral service, and getting everyone home safely. This was when it hit me the hardest. I was numb. I didn't want to go home but didn't know where else to go. Fortunately, or not, who knows, there was a brand new Ikea on the way home, and they are very good for wandering around and getting lost in, and I'd never even been to one before. Two hours later Eric called to make sure I was okay. I was.

Too Late*2011

I'd always get lost on the way to your house
Wait, I'm lost again, I'm turning around
I'm determined this time to figure this out
I've come too far to be turning back now

295 to 17 to 301 to 24
Turn right at Winn Dixie, stay left at the fork
Keep your wits about you
And call if you need me to wait
And you always knew I'd be late

I made a wrong turn, I'm going the wrong way
All I see around me are tractors and hay
Take the back roads through the country
So much faster, you'd always say

295 to 17 to 301 to 24
Turn right at Winn Dixie, stay left at the fork
Keep your wits about you
And call if you need me to wait
And you always knew I'd be late

I made it, I got it
You'd be so proud
I finally got it, I made it
It's just a little late now
I finally made it, I got it
I'm standing at your door
But there is no answer
Because you don't live here anymore

295 to 17 to 301 to 24
Turn right at Winn Dixie, stay left at the fork
295 to 17 to 301 to 24
But you don't live here anymore

No, you don't live here
Anymore

~*~

CHAPTER 12

It had already been decided that once dad passed, Tom was going to go live with our mother in Savannah. I helped him pack up a few things, drove him to the post office to ship a bunch of it, and said my goodbyes. My uncle was kind enough to drive him to the airport the day of his flight since I had to work. I tried to immerse myself in my new store and staff, and my new marriage, which I was quickly learning was the best thing that had ever happened to our dysfunctional relationship. Eric really loved me and turned out to be an amazing husband.

About four months later though, I was closing one night, and Leah called. As I think I've mentioned, my phone stays in my purse in the office but I check it every so often. She had called several times and left tearful messages about "I'm sure you've heard by now, but let me know if there's anything I can do for you." I had not heard. I called her back immediately and she informed me that Blair had died the night before. He was staying at a local motel because they had air conditioning and his apartment did not and it had been insanely hot the last few days, as in record-breaking late July in Michigan hot. The housekeeping staff found him that morning. They didn't know what he had died of, but it didn't look like drugs or foul play of any sort.

I lost it. I don't know how I got through the rest of my shift, but I let my staff know I'd just learned a very dear friend of mine was just found dead, and I'd like to get out as quickly as possible. They all kicked it in to high gear and gave me their hugs and support and were done in about twenty minutes after I locked the doors at closing time (even though it normally takes about an hour).

Fortunately, his service was held the following Saturday and I just so happened to be off that day. It was the most amazing event I've ever attended. You really kind of had to know Blair, but he was the kindest, most inspiring man I'd ever met. He was black and gay, and very proud of both of those traits and a big proponent to all kinds of groups and events for the furthering of blacks and/or gays, in addition, obviously to being a musician/writer/teacher. I only even mention this because I know he would want it known. I didn't even realize until everyone got up to tell their stories at his service that he had encouraged most of the local music scene to get up and play their first performance. I know he had done so for me. Hundreds of people met at the corner of Martin Luther King Blvd and Cass Avenue and we marched and danced and sang behind a New Orleans style jazz band for about a mile up the Cass Corridor until we reached the church on the corner of the street that also housed the apartment building where he was living when I first met him. I cried the whole way, but half out of sadness, and half out of how amazed I was at how beautiful the whole thing was, and how many people showed up to tell their own personal story of Blair. He touched so very many lives, and I know he would have been blown away by his own celebration of life.

Later that afternoon I had a very strange sensation come over me. We were standing in the church lawn with all of the other guests and it was about 105 degrees out. I got somewhat light headed and just sort of forgot what I was thinking about. I felt like I wanted to say something but I didn't know what I wanted to say or to whom I wanted to say it. I'd had quite a bit of coffee that morning, had walked over a mile in the hundred degree heat, and had very little water, so I just figured I was dehydrated. It went away within a few minutes.

This happened several more times over the next couple years, but it was usually when I'd had a fair amount of coffee. I found that if I just cut coffee out, it generally didn't happen. Working in a restaurant with free coffee and espresso available to me all the time though, I didn't make it through most mornings without a cup or two.

CHAPTER 13

About a month later, that itch to do anything besides working on cars came back to Eric, and he decided to go to the Specs Howard School of Media Arts at night, after a ten hour work day because he knew we couldn't afford for him not to work. I was fully supportive because I knew how much he hated wrenching and I never want to be the one to tell someone not to follow a dream. Have I followed any of my dreams? No. But that's because I never know what they are. I want him to figure out what makes him happy and while fixing high end cars is somewhat lucrative, it's not satisfying to him. He made it all the way through the year-long program with almost no one at work knowing. I was amazed. I almost never saw him, and he got very stressed out and was exhausted all the time and we fought about the pettiest things, but when he finished I was so proud. I cried like a proud mother at his graduation.

During much of this time, our house was also under construction. There was a tree in the front yard that someone had hammered copper spikes into, trying to kill it. I believe it was the next door neighbor, but I obviously never asked him. During a pretty bad storm one night, it fell on our house. I was closing that night and Eric called me at the store around 8pm to let me know. It was rooted in the city's side of property on the other side of the sidewalk, and they had already come out, chopped it to pieces and had it removed and gone by the time I got home at 10pm. We found out later they'd had previous complaints about the tree and requests to remove it that were never adhered to. I'm guessing this is why whoever it was took matters into their own hands, and I'm guessing why the city made it out so fast to remove it. All I know is that we didn't kill the tree, but it fell on our house.

Fortunately, we were just renting, so this was really the landlord's problem, but unfortunately for us, he decided to turn this into a major renovation. It was only the front porch that was damaged, but it had an awning area with roofing shingles, and apparently, you can never match roofing shingles, so the whole house needed a new roof. And hey, while we're at it, since the house is getting a new roof, this might be a good time to fix the ceiling in the mud room. And because some of the siding was a little gouged, why don't we re-side the whole house?! And then we'll replace the front door, and the side door, and of course it will need all new footing, and while all the mesh is off of the openings in the crawl space, a cat is going to make its home under your living room which Apollo will spend day and night sniffing the floor looking for! All while the landlord is trying to coordinate with his other two business partners, as well as the contractor, who was only present half the time. The fact that we weren't paying the contractor meant we were the last to know everything.

We had made it very clear to the landlord that if anyone was coming inside the house that we wanted to be home for that. He should have passed this on to the contractor, who should have passed it on to his men, but I came home from lunch with a girlfriend to men in the mudroom who had ripped off the ceiling and climbed in over the wall! I called Eric, he called the landlord, he called the contractor, and it was a hot mess. This is when we started getting pretty upset. We were paying full rent to live there, and we didn't feel like anyone cared about our privacy or wishes. They left the roof off and only a tarp covering the gaping hole in the mudroom ceiling that night, and it was winter in Michigan.

The landlord offered us a hundred dollars off the next month's rent because the roof was going in on a Sunday and the satellite dish had to be disconnected for a while, and you know by now that Eric loves his football. We probably would have consulted a lawyer, but by this point I had told the landlord to give the contractor my phone number, and I frequently had weekdays off so they were able to finish up the job quickly. Then, of course, the furnace went out, in February. The landlord had this replaced, a whole two days later. Then the tiles started falling off the wall in the shower. We couldn't get out of this hellhole fast enough. We found another house to move into and left with a full month on our lease, which we paid for because our deposit was a month and a half, and I ALWAYS get my deposits back.

CHAPTER 14

We moved into a house we found on Craigslist only a few blocks away for about 10% more in rent, but felt twice as big. Except for the kitchen, which I think was smaller than my studio apartment kitchen, but at least the fridge had an icemaker that worked most the time. When the landlord's assistant, Colleen, was showing us the house, she said the previous tenants had left because they'd just had twins and they were convinced there was mold in the house, but rest assured there was no mold. She also took us into the basement and showed us a puddle of water in the corner and said "yes, it leaks, but only in this corner." She continued to let us know that Wally, the landlord, was aware of the issue and they've done everything short of re-laying the foundation which he was not willing to do. We didn't think a little bit of water in the corner was a big deal, and we were way too eager to get out of our current predicament, so we signed the lease and moved in.

There was a tree stump on the side of the driveway in the back yard that I hated. I tried digging it out and just made a bigger mess of it. Eric had to help me with it and he likes to tease me about it every now and then because I asked our friends if I could borrow their chain saw. Fortunately for me, he said no once he found out why I was asking. This is not how you remove a stump, but I know that now. The toilet was also leaking when we moved in, but Wally sent his handyman by, Randy. Yes, Randy the handyman, which always reminded me of "Terry the Dairy Man" that would call Cosi every few days for our milk order, but that's beside the point. Randy came by a couple other times for minor fixes, like when the pretty stained glass panel fell out of the high garage window in the middle of the night barely missing my car. I always felt bad for Randy, but I don't know why.

It turned out that low and behold, the basement did leak much worse than we were lead to believe, especially during a heavy rain storm, and there was indeed mold because of it. However, Randy came by and spent two days cleaning each of the rafters in the basement with bleach, sprayed some protectant on them, they gave us a dehumidifier, and the mold did not come back.

Shortly after moving into this house I was transferred to a different Panera Bread location which was about forty minutes from my house, but right off the freeway. When I first got there it was just about all female. All six managers were female and most of the associates. There was a lot of estrogen floating around that store, and let's just say there was probably a catfight or two until one of the managers got transferred away. I got along with everyone, but I have no idea how some people put up with this one lady I won't name that was there long before I got there. She was a bitch, plain and simple; just a lazy, rude, horrible manager.

Over the first few weeks I was there, I think at least five people quit. I was really convinced it was me. Sherry, the General Manager of the store I had come from did everything by the book. Every single teeny tiny detail down to the last drop had to be exactly by Panera standards and would make certain you knew if you were doing something incorrectly. She was married to an auditor, and eventually became one herself, so I had a pretty good idea of the way things were supposed to be run, and this new store wasn't following half the policies. I had already made a promise to myself that I was going to wait at least a month before trying to change anything so that people could get to know me, learn that I am just a fun-loving, goofy girl that also happens to be a manager, so I was trying extra hard to be friendly and nice, but people just kept quitting. Two of them on two separate occasions actually came in, worked half their shift, went on break, and never came back! Both on my shifts. I kept asking the other managers if it was something I was doing and they all insisted that no, it was not my fault, but I still felt like it was. That store just had a higher turnover rate than I was used to because it was in a much nicer area where the kids don't really need to work. My other stores had a lot of more grown up associates, half of which with young families to feed.

I got used to this quickly though. Seemed like every other day we were hiring somebody new. Fortunately though, in some ways, I was responsible for the product. Ordering, inventorying, organizing, storing, rotating, labeling, etc...if it had to do with product in the store that was my job. If our food cost was in the gutter, that was, essentially, my fault. If it had to do with people, like interviewing, hiring, training, scheduling, firing, etc...that was Sandy's job. Obviously we helped each other quite a bit, but I think we were each glad the other was responsible for the other thing. I was the people manager for about a month at my previous store and I hated it.

A few months after I'd been there, we had a change in the guard and got a new GM, Don. He and Michelle, the current GM, just switched stores because each was much closer to the other's house. I don't want to imply here that Michelle didn't care about policies and procedures, but let's just say she didn't exactly enforce them. Don, on the other hand, he did. I think he knew at least as much as Sherry had, but was way more tactful in letting you know if you were doing something other than the Panera way. He was much more pleasant to work for and I learned a lot from him. I think Sandy did as well, as did Amy, Christine, and Stephanie, the shift leaders at the time.

A few months later, at the end of March, our lease would have been up on our newest house, but we decided to stay for the first time ever. Eric had not found a job in digital media anything and was getting no help from the school, even though they insist to every incoming student they're practically guaranteed a job upon graduation, and career services is amazing at helping people get them, but that's another story we'll just skip right over. After a lot of conversations and soul searching, he realized his true passion in life was still golf. He had loved working at Sawgrass in Florida, and had worked at Oakland Hills for most of his youth and teen years. He loved playing, and loved maintaining the courses, and had tried going to turf school in Florida, but couldn't get the funding at the time.

After many long talks, and weighing all the options, we determined that he would need to go to Rutgers in New Jersey because they had an accelerated program. All turf, all day, for ten weeks. Then, a ten month internship that he could do anywhere in the country; and then another ten weeks back at the school. The only way we could even almost make this work is that Andrea said I could stay with her while Eric was away at school, Apollo included, and Eric could even stay as well during the ten months in between if he managed to find an internship here. Once he had completed the program, we would find our own place again. I would stay in Michigan, working at my current Panera because even though there are several out there, the cost of living is much higher and there were definitely no apartments where all three of us could stay, that I could afford to support us in. So this was our plan for a month or so at the beginning of 2013, but the program didn't start until October. I explained our plan to Colleen, the landlord's assistant, and we were going to sign another six month lease, but she had some computer problem and said she'd send us the new lease the next month with our rent statement, and the end of April.

Easter Sunday fell on March 31st that year. I remember I wore these fabulous pink pants I had found at the local thrift store for two dollars that I had also worn on Valentine's Day. I was very accustomed to working holidays by now as I'd been doing it for years; and especially Sundays because one of the other managers wasn't available on Sundays because she was very involved in her church. I know it made Eric rather upset that I was almost never home to watch football with him, even though I had requested it a bunch of times, but that's just the way the cookie crumbles when you can't make your own schedule. So, I opened Easter Sunday, but honestly, Easter really didn't mean anything to me at this point other than an excuse to wear some bright pink pants that would have been questionable, as a manager, any other day of the year. I know I became very spiritual during my father's illness, and I am hardly an atheist or anything, but let's just say, I had lost a lot of my fire for the Christian ways.

I don't remember anything special happening on that day, or the Monday that followed. Tuesday, the second of April however, seemed like any other day when I went into work at ten. Tuesdays were double duty for the product manager as inventory had to be done by close, and the truck order had to be in by noon, so I was always scheduled ten until seven on Tuesdays, but I usually tried to get there early just to make sure I was done with my truck order early enough to get out on the line and help by lunch, which usually got going by 11:30am. This particular day was no different, and I was pulled away as soon as I was done preparing my order but hadn't entered it into the computer yet, to help put together a rather large call-in order. As soon as it was done, around 11:58am I was sent to the office to go submit my truck order.

About three quarters of the way through the order I

started getting very confused. I looked at my twenty ounce coffee cup, my second of the morning already, and just shook my head at it thinking I'd had too much coffee again. Then my fingers stopped responding to the signals my brain was sending them. I kept trying to hit the zero but would hit the one, or vice versa. I remember staring at my fingers and saying "one" and I would hit another number. Miraculously, at this moment, my husband happened to call the store, which he never ever did because he knew I couldn't really take personal calls at work, and it would have been a crime to call during lunch rush; and he usually just called my cell phone and left a message. When I saw his name pop up on the caller ID though, I answered. I also rarely answer the phone in the office because it's usually a phone in that needs to be rung up at the registers in the front of the store. I answered and he proceeded to tell me he was leaving work and going to the doctor because his leg was really hurting him. I don't remember responding. I don't remember anything else until I woke up in the back of an ambulance with the paramedic lady asking me "we just had Easter, can you tell me what month it is?" I had no idea.

CHAPTER 15

As it was later relayed to me, I had apparently had a grand mal seizure. I completely blacked out, was shaking so violently that I fell out of the chair and the dishwasher girl heard me fall, looked into the little window of the office door, and ran and got Sandy to come open the locked door, because only managers had keys to the office. Fortunately, there was usually an ambulance in our parking lot because they would use our wi-fi while waiting for a call, so they were already there. My husband kept trying to talk to me on the phone not knowing that I was seizing and apparently was getting frustrated that I wasn't responding because he thought I had just gotten distracted at work, and didn't care about his injury. He called my cell phone and apparently left me a rather rude message that he made me delete before listening to once he found out what was going on. He called the store back about ten minutes later and asked to talk to me and the associate put a paramedic on the phone who told him what had happened and where they were taking me. He got there before even I did.

I was still very out of it at this point but I remember such a sense of relief coming over me when I saw him at the hospital as they were wheeling me in. He just had this pained, worried look on his face, but it was also very tender and loving. And as soon as I was settled he gave me the biggest hug and kiss on the top of my head and didn't leave my side for hours. They did a few tests and determined I would be better suited at a bigger hospital so I was transferred a few miles over to a hospital I had delivered a whole lot of catering to while Kristen, the coordinator of my original Panera, was out on maternity leave.

Initial CT Scans and an MRI indicated I had a rather large brain tumor, but they didn't know what type yet, or whether it was malignant or benign. They scheduled the biopsy for Thursday morning. We called Andrea, my family, my job, Eric's job, anyone that might need informing. Eric's dad came by the hospital and got my keys so he and Karen could go get my car from my store, get into our house and pack us a bag and take Apollo to their house. I remember Andrea came to visit me in the hospital that night and brought pizza with her from one of Eric's favorite pizza chains, but it was terrible. I was also informed well after the fact that we watched the movie "Trouble with the Curve" but I don't remember that part, and apparently she was asked to leave halfway through because visiting hours had been over for a little while and we were making too much noise, but I don't remember that either. I don't really remember much of this hospital stay other than Eric almost never left my side, slept on a very uncomfortable looking waiting room sort of couch the whole time and barely ate. Sandy came to visit me at one point and insisted he go get something to eat because he looked terrible.

I really don't remember the day of the biopsy as I'm sure I was under a heavy amount of anesthesia for the rest of the day, but I do remember the flock of doctors that paraded through my room the next day. I felt like I met every doctor in the tri-state area. I was initially informed that there were actually two tumors and they were Astrocytoma, stage three. I imagine I was in shock, but I don't really remember feeling anything at this news. I just felt like "okay, so...what do we do about it?"

We were released the next day and had a slew of appointments lined up already. Several were with the neurosurgeon that had performed the biopsy so he could remove the staples and take a look at the wound. (Is it still called a wound when it's surgical? I googled it and apparently it is, but that just doesn't sound right to me.) The other few appointments were with the man that was slated to be my oncologist, Dr. Fata. I remember his office seemed way too nice. It was clearly brand new, freshly remodeled and had beautiful blue glass stones and fountains and fancy stuff that was nice to look at, but didn't feel like a doctor's office. I suppose this was the goal, but it gave me an odd feeling.

He ran some blood work and told me my iron was low and maybe my insurance would cover some shot treatment to boost it, but it was very expensive. Turned out my insurance did not cover it so I just started taking over the counter iron supplements. These were very constipating, as was the steroid I was now on. I was on all the same medicine my dad had been on, same steroid and same anti-seizure. Let me tell you, my dad never seemed to have any reaction whatsoever to his Decadron, the steroid, but I sure as hell did. It made me break out in horrible acne all over my chest and face, I was hot all the time, voraciously hungry all the time, and very cranky because of it. Nothing could satiate me. I was eating probably three or four times more than I had previously and gained over twenty pounds in a month, which is a lot for someone who only weighed 120 to begin with. And I didn't like to be touched anymore because I was just so hot and miserable. Eric stuck with me though, every step of the way.

It was apparently not the original plan to do a removal surgery. Dr. Fata wanted to start radiation and chemo right away, but Eric did a lot of research and wanted to talk to a doctor that would operate, and we were referred to the

University of Michigan Neurosurgery Department where Dr. Sagher worked, who specialized in awake surgeries. Apparently, they can numb the area they are working on while the patient is fully conscious so they can speak and let the surgeon know if anything starts being affected. (There are some very interesting videos online about this type of surgery; in my favorite one, the patient is playing a guitar!) He didn't want to do this with me however because my tumor was so large he didn't want to risk it. He was afraid there was too much pressure and when he opened the skull it would spring out to some extent and he wanted to make sure I was on a breathing tube if this were the case. I can't say I was disappointed about this.

We spent many hours discussing the possible side effects. Frankly, he was very surprised I didn't already show any signs. I had never had any trouble finding the right words, or any tingling feelings, or weakness on one side of the body or anything. The only symptom I'd noticed were the minor "episodes" I'd had several times over the last few years, which were determined to likely have been mini seizures, but I'd convinced myself it was all in my mind because my dad had just died of a brain tumor. It amazed me that no one seemed to think that was relevant. They all said things like "it's not genetic," and "it really is just a case of lightening striking twice," which I still have a hard time believing.

He explained that with the type of surgery he would be performing, in the area where the tumor was, I would not be able to speak for up to a month afterwards; that it would all come back eventually, but it may be a few days, or it could be a few weeks. It may come back gradually, or it might come back overnight. I would still be able to take care of myself and wipe my own ass, but we should probably have a system in place for communicating if I was tired or hungry, or wanted something because I would still need a lot of help. I made a very extensive set of note cards. The top one said "I love you!"

He also explained there were several blood vessels

running through the area, and if he did happen to nick one, there was a possibility I would have a stroke and most likely lose the use of my legs, which would be permanent. There was also of course, with all major surgeries, particularly those in the brain, the possibility that I might not wake up at all. I didn't need time to think about it though, I'd already made up my mind to have it done. We scheduled it for about two weeks out, April 24th.

We spent the next couple weeks training Eric how to take care of the bills and the banking and what the usernames and passwords to everything were, because this had all previously been my job. I made him extensive cheat sheets because I was very particular about how I liked to keep our bills and spending money organized, and how I paid each thing and why. He listened and adhered to most of it, and then came up with his own system which was different from my own, but I figured I needed to learn to let go of this and let him do it his way, which worked out just fine. It probably seems like I'm setting up to say he ruined our finances, but he didn't. It was a real "learning experience" for me. I also called everyone in my family to inform them they would probably not here from me personally for a while after the surgery, but Eric would keep my Aunt Jan informed and she would relay the messages if there was any news. I also started a blog at JenisProgress.blogspot.com (shameless plug) to let everyone know what was going on, and that I would be updating when there was news, and Eric would update it with the successful surgery results as I would not be able to.

We had to drive out to the university hospital a few times before the surgery for different blood work and what they call a "Live Mapping MRI," where the patient is actually involved in the MRI and they can determine what areas of the brain are used for what thought processes. I'm pretty good at lying perfectly still when I need to, but it was even more important for this one because I had to pay attention to images in front of my eyes and think certain things at certain times, and make my mind go blank at other times. Have you ever tried to make your mind go completely blank?! Impossible. It is for me anyway. The tech suggested to just think of a white table cloth, but I work in a restaurant, the image I got was a fine dining table with candles and flatware. I just tried to think of a white square. Then they would show me pictures of objects and I was supposed to say the word in my mind, but not mouth the word; and we had to repeat that part about three times, even though I am certain I was not mouthing the words. This went on for about two hours. I was getting kind of annoyed, which is hard to do to me, but eventually, we were done.

We decided to spend the night before the surgery in a hotel right around the corner from the hospital as it was about an hour from our house and we were supposed to be there by 7:30am. We got dinner at the Applebee's or Chili's or whatever it was across the parking lot. This was not the greatest idea because apparently Tuesday was kids' night and it was packed with families with small children. I know, I'm an ass and families with small children probably hate me and my people who don't like the sound of other people's children crying or shouting or whining, but I already work in a restaurant where I have to put up with it over fifty hours a week. I wanted what could potentially have been my last meal to have a little bit of peace, but no, this was not the place for it, and I had to stop eating by 8pm, so Applebee's or Chili's or whatever it was, is where it was going to have to be.

We woke up the next morning and went straight to the hospital and checked in. In less than an hour I was taken to where I could change into my gown and put all my personal items in a bag to give to my husband when I was taken in for surgery about an hour later. He was allowed to sit with me while we waited for the surgeon to come by and go over everything with me again, and the nurse to put the IV into my arm. The whole time we were talking and laughing and taking goofy pictures of me in my gown and cap. I'm sure I should have been nervous, but I'd had a really good feeling about this surgery. I'm not normally someone that "gets feelings" about things, but I just had a feeling, with no better way to describe it, that this was going to go well, so I wasn't nervous. I'm sure Eric was, but he hid it well. Eventually they came to put the anesthesia in my IV and obviously, I don't remember anything after that.

I am told the surgery took about six hours, which is what we expected. They gave Eric a pager and told them they would page him with updates. His father and my uncle came up to the hospital shortly after they took me in. I guess the surgeon spoke to him when I was out and told him everything seemed to go just fine, but I wasn't conscious yet so they didn't know for certain the extent of my ability to communicate. I do remember waking up though. The surgeon's assistant asked me "what is four times nine" and I *said* "thirty six." Aside from having the worst headache of my entire life, I was perfectly fine, able bodied, and even able to speak; which wasn't even supposed to be an option. I found out later that when the assistant texted the surgeon that I was "doing math," he thought she was kidding. He asked her how I was really doing and she told him she was serious.

I spent the rest of the day in the ICU and don't remember much of that because they were giving me morphine. If you're curious what type of surgery I had just google "Bifrontal Craniotomy." I warn you though, it's pretty intense. I had staples all the way across the top of my head when they removed the bandages, and to this day I can still tell where the metal plate is and where the bolts are holding it in place.

The surgeon came to visit me that afternoon and seemed very pleased with the surgery. He let us know that there was only one tumor, but it was about the size of an avocado, and he had removed about ninety five percent of it, but felt that the other five percent would be too risky, and that radiation would hopefully take care of that. I was pretty out of it for much of the next few days, which was amplified by the fact that I couldn't focus on anything because my face was so swollen I couldn't put my contacts in and my head was still too damaged to put my glasses on, and I am very blind without my vision aides. Eric watched the NFL draft next to me, and I mostly slept.

The first night was pretty bad. I'd had a urinary catheter in the whole day so I didn't need to get up to go to the bathroom, but apparently there is metal in it so it had to be removed for the follow up MRI I had to get at about midnight. As soon as I got back to the room I begged my night nurse to put it back because otherwise I was going to have to call her in at least every hour because I have an incredibly small bladder. She asked a doctor and they said no, but she was very nice about bringing me the bedpan probably every twenty minutes for the next hour. After the third time she checked my bladder and I was indeed retaining urine so she was able to do a temporary catheter or something to release most of the urine so that I was able to sleep, but my head hurt too badly to sleep much.

The next day I was moved out of the ICU to a room on the neurology floor, but with a roommate. There were curtains up between the sections of course, but she was always on the phone, or had her family visiting, or was snoring while she slept. I feel like we probably would have stayed another day, but after twenty four hours sharing a room with this woman, I decided I could be just as miserable at home on my couch as I could in the hospital, and I requested to be discharged, which took several hours. I'll never understand why there is always an intense hold up when a patient is ready to go home. It took even longer with my dad.

Eventually, the nurses had the prescriptions ready which fortunately included a gradual tapering off of the bloody steroid and had explained what I needed to take when to Eric, and we were sent down to the hospital pharmacy, which had one person working and a line of at least six people waiting. He parked me in my wheelchair off to the side and stood in line for a few minutes, but could see that I was still in a lot of pain and really wanted to get home, so we left.

We stopped at our local CVS pharmacy where I already filled all my other prescriptions and they had everything except for one thing that we had to go to another CVS for a few miles away. I just remember it was very bright that day and I couldn't put my sunglasses on so I just tried to keep the visor down and my eyes closed, but it still hurt pretty badly. Eventually, we had all the medication in the county and headed home. I'm pretty sure I went straight to bed, after wolfing down the McDonalds we had also stopped for.

Over the next few days I had good moments and bad. I really scared Eric one night because he was asking me questions and I would just look at him and kind of smile, but not answer the question, but this was only the second night after we got home, and it was very late, and honestly, looking back now, I think I was just really high. I had never really smoked before because I am a complete lightweight and it would just put me to sleep, but I've been told Marijuana is of great help to cancer patients, and it's medically legal in Michigan, if you have a card, which I do now, so every now and then when I'm nauseous or have a bad headache, I'll smoke, and it sure does help.

Eric, bless his soul, followed me around the house the first few days until he felt he should give me some space. On probably the fourth day home he was allowing me some private time in the bathroom when I started feeling lightheaded in the shower. I finished rinsing and turned around and shut the water off, and then I fell. I don't remember the fall, but I think my knees just buckled out from under me because I didn't topple over, I just went straight down and landed on my butt and snapped back to consciousness as Eric came bursting through the door asking "what happened" with that same pained but tender look on his face. I simply said "I fell."

I got out of the shower and wrapped up in a towel and sat on the toilet a few minutes until I felt better. After asking me at least twelve times if I was certain I hadn't hit my head, he decided we would not be running errands that day. He had our friend, Corrie, bring us some groceries because he didn't want to leave me alone and I was in no shape to be leaving the house. Fortunately, we had a bunch of friends offering to help us with whatever we needed. Corrie would not be the last.

CHAPTER 16

A week or so later we drove back out to Dr. Sagher's office to have the staples and sutures removed, and discuss further treatment and the pathology report. Turned out, it was really a stage 4 Glioblastoma Multiforme, exact same one my dad had given into just two years prior. Dr. Sagher said it was very unlikely they had anything to do with each other, but he would be willing to bet my tumor was already present and growing when he discovered he had his. Looking back, of course I wish I'd gotten checked out when I had those little episodes, but I had asked my dad's surgeon if my brother and I should get checked out and he said no, it's not hereditary, and my insurance at the time wouldn't have covered the CT scan, so I didn't. Like I said, I figured it was all in my head, for lack of another way to describe it. No pun intended, really.

Too Early*2013

She was born six weeks early
Weighing 5 pounds and 5 ounces only
The doctors with only her interests in mind
Said she can't go home yet, she must stay the night

Too early, too early
Too young and too fragile
Too early to go home

When she was just a child of 8
Her parents decided to separate
She chose to go live with her mother
Within months only, she wanted to go home
But selfish mother said no

Too early, too early
Too young and too fragile
Too early to go home

When she was only 29
And workin that unpaid overtime
The doctors found a mass in her brain
She had it removed and did all she could do
But it took her anyway

Too early, too early
Too young and to fragile
Too early to go home

Too early, too early
Too young and too fragile
Too early to go home

~*~

      After we were done with Sagher, he sent us to the other side of the hospital to meet Dr. Larry Junck, who would become my new Neuro-oncologist. He seemed like a very smart man, but had the personality of a potato. He explained that we would start radiation in several weeks, at which point I would also begin chemotherapy which would be taken in pill form an hour before the radiation. He explained that some people react poorly to chemotherapy and it tends to attack the white blood cells as hard as the tumor, so I would need to get my blood checked weekly because white blood cells make up the immune system. He also insisted I get a pneumonia vaccine before starting radiation and chemo. I feel like there was more because we were there for hours, but I think this is the bulk of it.

I know that when my second father, Don Milton, had cancer of the throat he drove out to Ann Arbor every day for his chemotherapy, but we really weren't trying to do that. We asked if there were any closer facilities and turned out the hospital about five miles from our house had a U of M Cancer Facility, so we scheduled an enrollment appointment there for about a week later.

This is where I met Dr. Abu-Isa, who became my Radiation Oncologist, and was much more pleasant to work with. He was younger and actually had a sense of humor. I filled out some more paperwork and scheduled my first day of radiation to be May 28th, the day after Memorial Day.

That weekend we went up north to Eric's dad's cabin on Hubbard Lake where we had been to several times before. I didn't normally love going up there for more than a few days because for whatever reason; I felt like life was going on without me. I don't relax well. I can't just sit still and do nothing. It makes me anxious, and there wasn't really much to do up there except sit around and drink, which is great for most people, but just not me. This time, however, I had no problem with it. The surgery had made me very passive and I was still not back to the normal me. I had no qualms sitting around doing nothing at this point, even though I couldn't drink because it would likely react poorly with my meds.

The day we left was the day before my birthday. We took the long way home which was very scenic. We stopped at the Tawas State Park which had a lighthouse and beaches and a gift shop, and Eric brought his fancy camera he had bought after graduating that took really high quality video and photographs and he took a whole lot of photos. There was also a dog friendly beach that we took Apollo to, but he hates water. He will not jump in the water unless he's chasing a favorite toy we've tossed in and as soon as he hits it he freezes, so he didn't want to go down by the water. We also stopped at a few little parks and piers on Lake Huron for more photos. It was quite lovely.

The next day Eric surprised me for my birthday. He said wear comfortable shoes and then blindfolded me and drove all over hell and gone trying to confuse me, but we really ended up at the zoo that was only a mile or two from our house. I love animals and had been asking to go to the zoo, but he never wanted to go because if he wasn't working, it was a weekend, and it was likely to be packed. But he wasn't working at this moment because I hadn't been given the okay to be left alone yet, and my 30th birthday happened to fall on a Monday. We walked all over, even though it was ridiculously hot for May 20th in Michigan. In typical Eric fashion, he took lots of incredible photos.

Later we went to Red Lobster for dinner, which is my favorite restaurant that we never go to because he's deathly allergic to seafood, but they have other things and made appropriate accommodations, as any restaurant should. I know it doesn't sound like much, but with Eric not working we were running out of savings quickly; so it was perfect for me. His birthday was five days later and our friends, Jeff and Aimee, who had just gotten married several days after my surgery, took us out to dinner at Eric's favorite local sports bar: 24 Seconds, in Berkley.

On Memorial Day we got together with my Grandmother and my Uncle at a restaurant on Woodward, where we had always met as a family, but no one knew why because no one really liked it all that much. My dad had always liked the giant goblets of beer they had. I think this is why I liked going, because it reminded me of my dad. My grandma and I talked about who knows what while Eric and my Uncle talked about cars and guy stuff. This was a typical gathering.

The next day I started my chemo and radiation. I was supposed to take the chemo one hour before the radiation began and couldn't eat for two hours before or after taking the chemo. I was told I might not need the anti-nausea pill I was prescribed so I didn't take it the first day. This was a mistake. On the way home from radiation I got very sick. I had to ask Eric to pull over and had the door open and was vomiting in the street before he even made it to the side of the road. When we got home I got sick again. I eventually took the anti-nausea and it went away, and I took it the rest of the week. I mentioned this to Dr. Abu-Isa when I met with him the next week, and he told me a lot of people experience bad nausea the first day, but then they were fine the following days. I didn't want to take the Zofran, the anti-nausea, because it was causing horrible constipation I thought I was done with now that I was off the steroid, so he prescribed a different, weaker anti-nausea called Compazine, which worked just fine to ward off the nausea once I discovered I needed to take it about an hour and twenty minutes before the chemo pill. And it did not cause constipation. Hallelujah! I know, probably more than you wanted to know, but I'm telling you, I wouldn't have included that if it weren't a very real problem.

Several weeks after I started the radiation my hair began to fall out. It itched like wildfire and they told me to use Aloe Vera and Aquaphor, but I couldn't really get it to the scalp because there was still hair in the way. Eric didn't want me to shave my head yet because he wanted me to wait and see just how much fell out because maybe I wouldn't need to shave it, and thought we should get a wig first because I might be self-conscious about having no hair (even though I had shaved my head twice before when I'd grown tired of my dreadlocks). Once enough had fallen out and it was clear I would not be able to just comb it over, we shaved it off and man did it help! I just thought it would make my scalp more accessible for the aloe, but it just stopped itching altogether.

I had done a lot of research on wigs, and already had a few from my performing days that I never wore, but turned out there was an American Cancer Society shop a few miles up the road that gave me one for free. They had a very limited selection and I didn't love the color, but I did like the style. It was synthetic so it held its shape even after washing. I also called my insurance company and it turned out they would reimburse me for a wig purchase if I had a prescription for a "cranial prosthesis" which Dr. Abu-Isa was happy to write for me. If I was going to wear it to work it had to be human hair because synthetic would melt if I got near anything too hot and between the bagel toaster, the Panini grills, the soup well and the rethermalizer, not to mention the giant rack oven that was usually at 420 degrees to bake baguettes all day; staying away from heat sources was not an option. So one Saturday we went to the local beauty supply store that our friend, Julie, had recommended as having quite a wide selection and helpful staff and tried on probably a dozen before settling on one that was my second favorite, but my first favorite just didn't fit right.

The next weekend I wore one of them Saturday, when we met Brad and Julie at a park by our house to watch Brad and the crew of Julie's new show, "Low Winter Sun" play softball. It was very hot this day and they kept losing players, so by the third game, Eric was playing. The next day I wore the other one to a Detroit Tigers game that Eric's work bought out the Pepsi Porch for, something they do every year, but it was even hotter this day and we had no seats, only the bleachers in direct sunlight so we stayed an inning or two and then went home to watch the rest of the game inside. Normally, I love the hot weather, but I was still coming off of the steroid, and taking chemo every day, so I really did not have the energy to keep walking around the concourse where it was cooler. Problem was, my hair was still falling out and I was still getting radiation to my head, so my scalp was very tender and wigs were very uncomfortable, so I didn't wear either one again for quite some time.

During these few months it was also a constant administrative struggle with the disability company. Thank the Lord I had even added disability to my policy at the beginning of 2013 because it was only a few dollars per check, but man was it a headache filling out all the necessary forms and having the doctors sign off and fax it over and they needed updates every other day it felt like and if the administrative assistants at the radiation place didn't fax something over, or the disability company didn't get it, my payments were delayed, which were only sixty percent of my salary to begin with, and now I had to mail in checks to Panera to pay for my insurance premiums up front because they couldn't deduct it from my check anymore. I was also having a hard time with the Social Security Administration in the beginning as well, but fortunately, it eventually all got sorted out; after many many hours of my indefinite amount of time left in this world on the phone with everyone and their neighbor's cousin. I must also input here that my aunt Jan in particular, but also a few others, did offer to help with this element, but I declined. As big as a pain in the neck that it was, honestly, I didn't have anything else to do, and I need to always have something to do. I wasn't even allowed to drive because the chance of seizure was still eminent.

About a week before the end of my radiation treatments, in early July, I started to itch. Not incredibly bad, but all over my body and with no sign of rash or dry skin. It would move around and no amount of scratching would really satiate. I asked every one of my doctors: oncologists, nurses, physician, even gynecologist, and no one had an answer. I tried every possible anti-itch solution under the sun, but only a few seemed to do anything at all. This went on for many months.

CHAPTER 17

At the end of the six weeks of radiation, I had a month off. Unfortunately, this is when I scheduled all my other appointments I couldn't have while in treatment, like my root canal I had canceled way back in April. I know most people would never expect to hear these words, but man was I happy to get that done. That tooth had been bothering me for years! I also had my yearly physical (for the first time since I needed one for summer camp when I was thirteen) and my annual visit to the lady doctor.

I also had a very nice trip down to Georgia to visit my mother and her whole side of the family. My grandparents live in a lovely retirement community about an hour outside of Atlanta now, and my mother is only several hours away so she and Tom drove to Atlanta, picked me up at the airport and then we all went to my grandparents' place. My Aunt Jan even flew in from California on an airline credit she had from a flight she'd missed earlier in the year. She is one of the most open-minded, enjoyable people I have ever met and I'd only seen her once for a few hours probably five years prior when she was in town for a high school reunion and before that, not since the summer after my freshman year of college, so at least another five years.

It was lovely to see everyone. I only stayed for a few days, but it really was nice to get away for just a few days and see Georgia, my second favorite state. While I was down there, Eric called me one morning to let me know that Dr. Fata, my original Oncologist, the one with the fancy brand new office, had been raided by the FBI the night before and it was all over the news in Michigan. Apparently, the expensive Iron supplement shot he had said I needed, he recommended this to everyone, even if their iron wasn't low. He also continued treating cancer patients even after their window of life was clearly closed; or what's worse, he continued treating patients who were in remission and didn't need chemo or radiation at that time! He didn't think we should do surgery on me because it was "too dangerous." He was just going to start chemo and radiation right away, which is why Eric had insisted on a second opinion and we were referred to Dr. Sagher. In Dr. Sagher's professional opinion, I probably would have died before the chemo or radiation had a chance to do anything if we hadn't operated. This made me sick to my stomach. It still sends me into a silent rage just thinking about this asshole that was perfectly happy to just let me die for his own profit. I am usually a kind, compassionate, caring person, but this man, who...............I just hope he's being violently violated in some prison somewhere. What a giant bag of xxxxxx.

Deep breaths. Anywho, I had a nice month off of cancer, in a sense. I still had to take my anti-seizure medicine, but otherwise, I was treatment free for one month until my first post chemo and radiation MRI to create a new baseline, as it was explained to me. This was on August 9, 2013. Guess what the results were? It was clear! The radiation and chemo had apparently knocked out the other five percent of tumor that Dr. Sagher didn't feel comfortable removing. Dr. Junck, my oncologist, told me the scan looked about as good as it could for this stage of the game. We would begin what is called "cyclic Temodar" for twelve months. I would take Temodar, the chemo pill, at a much higher dosage for five days of every four weeks. This time, I would take it at bed time. We were able to pick up the first cycle at the hospital pharmacy that day.

Towards the end of the month, two friends and former co-workers, Kristin and Lisa, threw me a giant benefit. Eric did not love the idea, but I cleared it with him first, and he also spoke to a trusted friend that told him "sometimes you have to let people help you." It really was beautiful. It was a silent auction at Champps, the sports bar that Andrea went to all the time that Dwayne, Kristin's husband, worked at. Kristin and Lisa did such a phenomenal job getting donations from restaurants, spas, stores and other businesses and promoting to get so many people to attend, that it was such a huge success. I even brought a few pieces of my own artwork, which did not get bid on; but Lisa, who was a painter and had donated a few of her own pieces, and I exchanged work. Her painting, which reminds me of Birch trees, is on my living room wall right now.

The first cycle was symptom free. I took my Compazine, the low-grade anti-nausea about forty five minutes before the Temodar, and had no issues. The second cycle we drove an hour back to Ann Arbor to pick it up at the hospital pharmacy because no local pharmacy carries it, and we were informed that my insurance was not going to cover it. We spent hours on the phone in the hospital basement right outside the pharmacy trying to figure out why they had allowed it the month prior, but no one could tell us. Apparently, my insurance flat out requires I get my Temodar from a certain mail-order pharmacy called Curascripts. For whatever reason, my blood work, white blood cell count, was not high enough that I could even start cycle two for another week anyhow, but it was still a very frustrating wasted trip.

October 4, 2013 I had my second post chemo and radiation MRI, which also came back clear. We were also still having follow-up visits with Dr. Abu-Isa at this time. I had an appointment with him about ten days later where I asked him to feel the back of my head where I was convinced I felt bumps that were excruciatingly itchy. He said he didn't feel anything underneath the half inch of hair I had grown back by this point, but I was certain. I didn't push it too hard because at this point, I'd been itching for four months and no one had a suggestion, so honestly, I just accepted it. Dr. Junck's office also told me I needed to get a flu shot, which I was very torn on, but I got it and I did not get the flu. Thank God.

Tuesday, October 22 is when I got my flu shot and when the Temodar was ordered from Curascripts. When a prescription is ordered through Curascripts, it has to "process" for twenty four to forty eight hours and then they call the patient to schedule delivery, which cannot be done before it has finished "processing." When I hadn't received a call by Thursday, I called them and they informed me they had called me four times over the past twenty four hours, calls I never received, because they had a question. They were out of the brand name, would the generic be okay? I told them I didn't see why not, but I would check with my doctor and let them know, which God knows why they didn't just contact the doctor. The next morning I called Dr. Junck's office and confirmed the generic would be just fine and called back Curascripts. This was now Friday morning. Saturday morning I called them yet again to try to schedule delivery but there was still some problem and I was told I would receive a call back. Eventually Eric got involved, spoke to a supervisor and her supervisor, and eventually Monday we scheduled it for overnight delivery for Tuesday. The brand name Temodar showed up.

I was scheduled to start that night, cycle three now. I didn't expect any issues, but this first night I had a horrible allergic reaction to the medication, even though it was the exact same I'd been taking since May. The worst part of it was that about a half hour after I took it I got this ferocious burning sensation all over my entire body. The best analogy I can think of is that it felt like thousands of tiny matches trying to poke their way through my skin from the inside, all over my entire body, with the worst of it inside my vagina. It was excruciating! I had never had an allergic reaction to anything before, so I didn't know what this was. It went away after about forty minutes.

Then, about two hours after I took the Temodar, just as I was about to drift off to sleep, my throat started to close up. I could still breathe fine, and I could still swallow just fine so I wasn't too worried about it, but this is what clued me in to the fact it might be an allergic reaction. I took a couple Benadryl, but about five minutes later I got crazy nauseous and immediately threw up. I spent the rest of the night dry heaving because there was nothing left in my stomach. This was one of the worst nights of that year. I slept on the bathroom floor for about twenty minutes at a time.

The next four nights I did not get sick, but I did get the horrible burning sensation just as bad. I wish I had realized it was an allergic reaction, but I just didn't. For five straight nights I just put up with tiny matches. It was really rather terrible, but I dealt with it. I wish I could say it got better as the cycle went on, but it did not.

Several days later I got a rash on my stomach, around November 6. This was particularly itchy at moments. Not consistently, but when it itched, oh buddy, did it itch. We went out to Pittsburgh to visit our friends, Julie and Kase, who we had met in Florida, but Julie had moved back home to Pittsburgh before we'd moved back home to Detroit. It was only about a five hour drive and I'm surprised we hadn't gotten together sooner. We went to the Detroit Lions vs. Pittsburgh Steelers game, which the Steelers won handily. It was pouring. Rained the whole game. We went to the Hofbrauhaus afterwards, and I remember my stomach itching horribly. I had to excuse myself to the restroom, but again, no amount of scratching would satiate the itch. There seemed to be weeks that didn't itch as bad as others, but I wasn't keeping very good track, so in my mind, I was convinced it was related to my birth control which had changed a few times over the past few months for various reasons.

The last day we were in Pittsburgh as we were slowly packing up to get back on the road, the girl we had asked to watch our dog called to ask where he might go if he got out. There had been a very bad storm the night before, which had hit Detroit as well, and the gate blew open. She checked that it was closed when she let him out around 6am, but when she let him out again about 9am before leaving for work, it had blown open. I'm sure it took incredible guts for her to call us and let us know, but I'm super glad she did. Fortunately, I had just the past week walked up to the pet store and happened to get him a customized collar tag with his name and my phone number, but I was still terrified he'd get hit by a car before a concerned citizen found him. We threw everything in the car and were about to start speeding back home when she called to say she found him and everything was just fine. He was only a block away, playing in a pile of leaves, and he came running as soon as he saw her and jumped right in her car. I'm not going to lie though, those ten minutes probably stole years from my life. This was the first time I had even an inkling of what my father was probably feeling the night I had walked up to my camp seventeen years ago. I wished I could have apologized some more to him for that.

We finished our coffee and said our goodbyes and planned for them to come visit us around the following March or April and we headed home. Several days later my chest broke out in an itchy rash. At the end of the month I started cycle four, which went exactly as the last cycle had: violently ill the first night, and evil burning sensation all five nights.

On December 9, 2013 I finally scheduled a dermatologist appointment because I finally had something of note to show a skin doctor. She said it was very likely not a drug related rash. Those are normally over the entire body, not just small, concentrated areas. She took a look at my abs and my chest, and took a little biopsy to send off to the lab, and gave me a prescription for a topical cream. This same day I developed the same rash on my left arm.

The next day I had my third MRI, which also came back clear. I had a follow-up appointment with Dr. Junck where I mentioned the new symptoms to the Temodar, to which he suggested Benadryl, two to start, three if I thought I needed it. Three turned out to be necessary, but also turned out to pretty much take care of the horrible sensations. He also prescribed a now third anti-nausea that I only took on the first night of the cycle, but it seemed to do the trick, for at least the next few cycles.

I had a follow up appointment with the dermatologist on December 19, 2013 where she determined it was "Folliculitis," inflammation of the hair follicle, and she prescribed a different cream and a foam, one for morning and one for night. These seemed to do the trick for a week or so, but the damned itching just came back. It always did.

We had a wonderful Christmas, despite itching and chemo. My Aunt Jan was waiting in the parking lot at a Walmart in California earlier in the month to get one of my nephews an Xbox One, which Eric really wanted and I could not find one anywhere, so when I mentioned this, she offered to see if she could get two. I jumped at the chance, expecting to pay her back, but she wouldn't let me. It showed up the week before Christmas. My computer had been overheating and having major CPU issues that we really didn't have the money to fix, so with the money saved from the Xbox One, Eric bought me a Surface 2, which was equally as difficult to find, but we eventually got one a few days before Christmas. On Christmas day our friends Brad and Julie came over, I cooked, and we all ate and drank and played silly board games. New Year's was even less eventful. At least we stayed up until midnight, but we didn't go anywhere or have anyone over. I had just completed a chemo cycle the night before.

CHAPTER 18

In the new year I ran into a brand new set of issues. As I had feared, I was now back at zero dollars spent as far as my insurance company was concerned. My itching was getting so bad it was keeping me up at night. I wanted to give the cream and foam ample time to do their thing before scheduling another dermatologist appointment though.

On Wednesday, January 15, 2014, Phil, the nurse/administrative assistant from Dr. Junck's office was supposed to have sent in the prescription for my sixth cycle of chemo. When I still hadn't received a call from Curascripts to schedule delivery by Friday, I called him back and oops! He hadn't sent it yet, but he promised he would send it before leaving for the day. The next day I called Curascripts and yes, they had received it, but it was still "processing." I called back later and turned out it was ready to schedule but was going to cost me $1300! Monday morning I called Phil back and he gave me some numbers to some assistance programs. He also took it upon himself to send the prescription to the hospital pharmacy, which wanted to charge me $1400, and would require payment up front, and I still don't think my insurance company would have allowed me to get it there, as they had not in the past. I didn't know all this at the time though and when I called

Curascripts back that night, they told me they could not send it to me because the hospital pharmacy already had an approved claim on it. I needed to call them and have them reverse the claim, but of course, they were already closed. Why wouldn't they be?

I called them first thing in the morning the next day and asked them to reverse the claim, but also explained that maybe it got sent to them in the process of the hospital social worker trying to help me. The pharmacist said she would check with the social worker and get back to me in forty five minutes, which of course, she did not. Several hours later I called the hospital pharmacy back and just had them reverse the claim so Curascripts could actually ship it to me, but it still took them another twenty four hours of "processing" before they could schedule delivery. It finally showed up the following Friday, the 24th of January.

This entire week my rashes were getting worse. It had spread across my chest, my left shin, and then my right ankle. The abs rash had gone away, thankfully, but the rest were terrible. I had a third dermatologist appointment on January 27. At this one she prescribed an antibiotic and now a third topical cream. She was still convinced it was folliculitis, despite some suggestions I had come up with, but what do I know? I'm not a doctor, or dermatologist or anything. I have a Fine Art Degree I've never used. The next day I started my sixth cycle, which went generally unnoticeable, aside from some marked fatigue, but I blame the Benadryl for that.

Fortunately, I was approved for both assistance programs I was referred to, the ACT Program, and the Musella Foundation for Brain Tumor Research, which helped me cover the ridiculous co-pays for my Temodar. I had a fourth dermatologist appointment on February 19, where she took yet another little biopsy and told me she would call me on Friday when the results came back. She did not. I called Monday to check the results and see if I should stay on the anti-biotic, but she was on vacation. Apparently my results came back negative for both the things she was testing for, but they swore they'd have her call me when she returned. I called two more times the next week, but never got in touch with the doctor. Miraculously however, the itching and rash finally went away. Hallelujah!! After eight treacherous months, it just went away one day towards the end of February.

The following month I decided to volunteer at the zoo the following summer because I was getting stir-crazy-cabin-feverish. We had the snowiest winter in Michigan history, and I was trapped inside the house for days as Eric was back to work full time now, had been for months, and it was way too cold out to be walking or riding my bike anywhere. I had an orientation on March 22, 2014 which Eric dropped me off at. I was referred by my grandmother on my dad's side as she had volunteered there a few years. I decided to be a "Zoo Ambassador" which basically stands at the front gate welcoming guests to the zoo or walks around and answers questions. The uniform consists of khaki's and a red zoo shirt. I detest khaki's. They don't look good on any woman. Women, am I wrong? I tried on twenty different pairs before just picking the least offensive pair that still didn't fit right.

April 2, 2014, Eric took the day off of work to celebrate my one year anniversary. We got a great deal on some great seats at the Detroit Tigers baseball game, which we won. I painted a nose and whiskers on my face, and video-bombed the couple in front of us when they were up on the big screen. We had a great time and I felt very much alive and healthy.

CHAPTER 19

This, my lovelies, brings us to current day. I am still on medical disability, but hoping to return to work when I'm finished with my cycles in August. I'm planning on volunteering at the zoo for most of the summer. I've been working on this book for the last few months so that I'd have a project to get me through the winter. My doctors tell me I'm doing wonderfully, and all my family and friends are amazed by my positive attitude. The doctors like to remind me however, not to get my hopes up, that the survival rate is extremely low. I've just passed my one year anniversary. I am convinced, however, that I have more to do. I don't know what that is yet, but I know it's out there to be discovered. It's like an adventure. A treasure hunt, if you will. One day I will figure out the pot of gold at the end of my rainbow. Until then, I will keep making art and music and riding my bike around the neighborhoods, and loving my husband and my dog and my friends and family, who have shown me nothing but love and support. I really don't think I'd have even made it this far without their love and support.

Let us hope and pray I write a sequel to this little novella.

This is my story to date.

This is not the end of my story.

To be continued...

93507026R00094

Made in the USA
Lexington, KY
15 July 2018